Intermittent Fasting for Women

Use One Meal A Day (OMAD), Water Fasting and Alternate Day Fasts for Diabetes, Insulin Resistance, Hormone Reset and Autophagy to Reverse Aging and Heal Your Body

Stacy Shaw

Table Of Content

Introduction

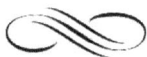

The search is on! It has been on for a long while now. Men and women alike have been on a quest to discover the fastest, shortest, and most effective means of losing weight, getting fit and staying healthy without necessarily undergoing surgery or any other major medical procedure. This quest has led humans to develop several methods of dieting and controlling eating habits that are mainly aimed at weight reduction.

Some of these methods have been effective, others, not so much. As a matter of fact, many dieting programs do not work, plain and simple! They are just another means of leading the unsuspecting public down a path that leads nowhere, fast! Some of these programs are very strenuous, rigorous, and cumbersome. This has made a lot of people give up on them, and even when they truly want to stick to the programs, they end up cheating due to the unrealistic nature of the diet programs.

Yet, others stick to programs they should have given up on long ago. They stayed on because of obsession and pressure – pressure to look and feel like others. Weight loss is an obsession for some (especially women).

A lot of women find themselves in this category because of the tendency of the female body to easily put on extra flesh here and there. It is easy for women to become obsessed about weight loss and jump at every diet program out there – and boy! there are really lots of dieting programs crawling around especially on the internet. The question is; how do you determine which is right for your body and which one actually works? The answer lies in due diligence. If people will diligently study for just a little bit, it will become obvious that there a few good programs that actually work and can suit them perfectly.

One of such programs is intermittent fasting. However, intermittent fasting is not entirely focused on weight loss. It is no diet at all; neither is it a way of starving yourself or going hungry for longer periods in order to lose weight! This book is written to bring to light the many health benefits of intermittent fasting, plus possible side effects and how to know if it is a good fit for you. If it is good for you, then you can use it as a way of life – a lifestyle.

You may know of people who swear by intermittent fasting; insisting that it works. You may also know others who have had less than pleasant experiences with this "cycle of eating and not eating". This book about intermittent fasting is not written from the angle just to suit the rave of the moment. On the contrary, this book is an honest attempt to present an unbiased and balanced view about intermittent fasting – its pros and cons.

This book is written with women in mind – women whose interest is not just on medical jargons or scientific terminologies; but whose interest is to find a tested program that truly works. I do not promise that intermittent fasting will work for you. What I do promise however is that this book will help you to know if intermittent fasting will work for you or not.

Even though this book was written specifically with the woman in mind, men are sure to benefit from the many useful tips, dos and don'ts that characterize this book. It is my hope that at the end of reading this book, you would have gathered enough facts to help you along your journey to stay fit and healthy.

Aside from weight loss, there are reports of lowered blood sugar, possible reversal of Type 2 diabetes, and activation of autophagy, plus lots of other health benefits derived from intermittent fasting. In this book, you will find safe methods, useful tips, and brilliant insights that will help improve your general health even if intermittent fasting is not for you.

The effects of fasting on the female hormones,

aging, metabolism, and stressor triggers shall be highlighted in this book. We shall also take a look at a few of the popular myths and misconceptions about intermittent fasting and take them down one after the other.

It is time to put the skepticism aside. It is time to get a clearer understanding of this type of fasting. I welcome you to study this material with an open mind to find out if it is meant for you. And for those who decide that intermittent fasting is for them, I will not hesitate to recommend that they seek proper medical advice from their healthcare provider before embarking on any type of fasting.

Chapter 1: Intermittent Fasting: What It Is

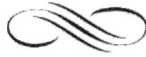

I magine, for a minute, that your good old pressing iron has no thermostat (the small device inside the pressing iron that regulates the temperature). You'll have to keep an eye on the pressing iron constantly to regulate the temperature by yourself. But the thermostat does the job of cutting off the temperature when it is too high or turning on the heat when the temperature becomes too low (according to the heat level you set the control lever). All this temperature monitoring happens without much of your attention as you use the pressing iron.

Now let's apply this analogy to you and food. You'll most certainly agree that eating nonstop is not only impracticable but also not in the best interest of your health. There is a natural thermostat (so to speak) that regulates your food intake. It does this to balance your fed state and your unfed state. Fasting is the natural thermostat that regulates our food intake.

We all do fast one way or the other. As a matter of fact, we do fast daily although not everyone does this by choice. When you have your breakfast, you are actually breaking your fast! The fast you started the previous night.

But intermittent fasting does not simply refer to the period of non-intake of food while you are asleep at night. If that were the case, and since everyone does that, there wouldn't be a need for this book, nor would there be a need for all the researches carried out on the subject.

I have said all of the above to say that intermittent fasting is the deliberate act of not eating for a certain amount of time even though you are hungry and have food to eat. The amount of time for fasting is entirely up to you. Also, which foods you choose to eat when you break your fast is entirely up to you. Intermittent fasting does not cover types of food to eat or not to eat; rather it focuses on when to eat and when not to eat. However, it is only common sense to keep to healthy foods at all times and especially during intermittent fasting.

It is perfectly okay to drink water or other liquids during fasting as long as the liquid does not contain calories. (If you are fasting for religious purposes, kindly lookup your particular system of belief for what is allowed during fasting. This

book does not give any suggestions in regard to religious fasting). It is also okay to take supplements that do not contain calories during intermittent fasting.

There have been claims and counter-claims about the health benefits (or otherwise) associated with intermittent fasting, but it appears that whether or not it will be beneficial depends largely on each individual. As we are unique individuals with different existing medical conditions and differing levels of hormonal balance, it will be quite difficult to say that what works for one applies to all.

It also appears that fasting and its benefits tend to work better for the male than for the female,especially with prolonged fasting. The normal workings of the female hormone may be thrown off balance during intermittent fasting but then again, individual differences cannot be ruled out. All of this notwithstanding, I will give some space, albeit briefly, to highlight the benefits of intermittent fasting. But first, let's take a quick look at what intermittent fasting is not.

What It Is Not

Is this not the same as starving? Am I suggesting that starved people do actually enjoy health benefits from starving?

No. Intermittent fasting is not starvation. And I am not suggesting there is any health benefit that can be derived from starvation. There is one huge difference between fasting and starving; choice.

When you fast, you have food and a choice to

eat, but you deliberately choose not to eat. You have a choice about when to eat and when not to. But starving means you have no choice about eating because, even though you are willing to eat, there is no food. When you fast, you may be hungry but you simply won't eat because you choose not to. But when you are starved, you are hungry but you can't eat because there is nothing to eat.

Some experts have also described intermittent fasting as alternating circles of eating and fasting. While I may want to agree with that, a keyword or phrase is still lacking in that definition or description. We all alternate between eating and fasting – at least we do so at night when we are asleep or even during our waking hours when we are not eating.

For it to be considered fasting intermittently, there must be a sense of deliberateness in the withdrawal from food and such withdrawal should keep to a predetermined number of hours.

So when you go to bed around 10pm for example and you did not eat until the following day around 7am before having breakfast, we could loosely say that was fasting for 9 hours. However, you will have to do better than that if you intend to derive any reasonable health benefit from the use of intermittent fasting.

Why Should You Fast?

What about hunger? How do you handle hunger during fasting? In fact, why should you go without food in the bid to get healthier? Isn't that counterproductive? Isn't food meant to keep us healthy?

The polar bear, crocodile, lungfish, and snakes among others, have something in common; they can go for months and sometimes years, without eating! It could be argued that certain animals are built for that, and that would be correct. But "*a human can go for more than three weeks without food — Mahatma Gandhi survived 21 days of complete starvation*" (Spector, 2018, n.p.).[1]

Now, don't get me wrong. I am not advocating that you go for prolonged periods without food. I am only stating the obvious: you have the ability to go for longer periods without food than you would normally do. And there is nothing "out of place" with fasting. Throughout history, humans have been fasting; sometimes because there was famine and sometimes for special reasons like spirituality or for religious reasons.

If you are completely new to the idea of fasting, the fear of going without food for longer periods than you normally would may cause you to be hungrier than you should. But with a little bit of practice, your body will get used to it. As a matter of fact, your body is designed to handle hunger for longer periods than you have been led to believe. There is a backup or reserve of energy your body taps into when there is no food in the primary food storage. But we shall discuss this a bit more when we talk about how intermittent fasting works.

Obviously, food is meant to keep us healthy; however, there are some changes – good changes – that occur in our bodies when we fast. They may also be a noticeable decrease in our blood sugar level and other changes in hormones. We shall get into the details of that later in the book.

Some people fast because they want to lose weight. There are indications that suggest that intermittent fasting may lead to weight loss due to fewer intakes of calories and the fat that is used up during the periods of fasting.

And the idea of saving time may be appealing enough to make some people consider fasting every once in a while. I mean, considering the time it takes to prepare a good meal three or more times in a day, and the time it takes to clean up after eating, it wouldn't be such a bad idea to fast after all. And then throw into the mix the money you'll save. Now that's some motivation too!

The truth of the matter is this, fasting isn't as difficult as it may appear. You already go some hours every day without food; intermittent fasting is simply extending those hours a little bit more. It's really that simple.

How It Works

Alright, let's take a quick look at how intermittent fasting works. Let's see the science behind it.

When you eat, your body converts the food into energy in sugar form and stores it in your liver. The hormone called insulin is in charge of storing the ingested sugar to be used later. Insulin level increases when you eat to help the body store up the energy ingested. But our livers have a limited storage capacity, so when we eat, the liver can only hold as much sugar or glucose before it is filled up. The good news is that there is an alternate storage for the spillover of energy ingested. It is stored up as body fat which has unlimited storage capacity. In essence, your body has two energy storage; the liver which is easily accessible, and body fat which is a bit less accessible.

Now when you eat, your body is busy digesting the food, breaking it down, and ingesting and extracting nutrients and energy. When you stop eating your body takes a little break from all that work and concentrates on using the energy to keep you going. This is where fasting comes in. When you are not eating, your body can use up the excess energy stored up as fat to sustain you. In other words, fasting burns up fat stored in the body. This happens because when you do not eat, your insulin level drops. This drop in insulin level sends a signal to your body to start using up or burning up energy stored as fat since energy is not coming from food at that moment.

Basically, your body is either in a state of high insulin – that is, when you are fed – or in a state of low insulin – when you fast. It is either you are accumulating energy from eating or you are burning it up. The healthy state of being would be to find a balance between the two states. Finding this balance ensures that there is no overall weight gain.

Intermittent fasting, when done in moderation is not injurious to health. There is enough body fat for your body to "feed itself" when you are not feeding it by eating food. The key is to strike a balance between eating and fasting. Eating continuously (is that even possible?) or eating for the most part of your day may lead to weight gain when done over a long period because your body has not had any time off to burn the energy you provide for it.

It is, therefore, a wise practice to interject eating with safe amounts of hours of not eating. The purpose of storing energy is so that it will be used up. So allow your body to do what it was designed to do perfectly. It is safe for animals; it is also safe for humans.

A quick word about intermittent fasting: please be sure to consult a medical expert if you are pregnant or lactating before embarking on fasting. If you are on any blood sugar medication for diabetes, please do ensure to consult a qualified medical expert to adjust dosages or to determine if you are fit for fasting. Generally, if you have any pre-existing medical condition, please consult your healthcare practitioner for advice before practicing intermittent fasting.

Intermittent Fasting: The Back-Story

The idea of intermittent fasting and its benefits are not as new as we would want to believe. Long before modern civilization, hunter-gatherers practiced intermittent fasting because food in its various forms, and agriculture as we have today, wasn't discovered back then. Basically, since hunter-gatherers do not get a kill every single day, they had to "ration" their kill and go without food for longer periods until such time when they are able to find food. Their bodies adapted to this form of eating pattern and they were healthy – lean, strong, and very active. Evidently, they were unknowingly enjoying the benefits of intermittent fasting.

Very dated evidence shows that the ancients in Egypt, Greece, and Indy, practiced intermittent fasting to prevent some types of diseases as well as treat them.

Some very early traditions such as the Native

North Americans usually practiced a type of fasting that is done throughout the tribe to ward off threats of disasters.To appease their gods, the Incas, as well as the Native Americans of Mexico,practiced fasting also. *"Fasts were also part of the fertility rites in primitive ceremonies. Many of these ceremonies were held at the vernal and autumnal equinoxes and survived for centuries"* (Microsoft Encarta, 2008, n.p.).[2]

Various religions of the world also encourage fasting as a way to "discipline" the body to show contrition or repentance. It has the benefit of instilling self-control in adherents (and other health benefits too, although this may not be their focus). This practice is as old as the various religions themselves.

The "day of atonement" or "Yom Hakippurim," is a type of fasting practiced in Judaism. The 40 days Lent is a period of fasting observed annually by Roman Catholics to commemorate the period of fasting observed by Jesus. Ramadan is a fasting period extending for between 28 to 29 days observed in Islam.

The point of all this is to show that fasting has been with us for longer than many people realize. It is not a strange or new practice.

In more recent times, intermittent fasting began to gain popularity through the media as more and more documentaries, health publications, and books began highlighting the benefits of the practice especially as it relates to weight loss. Prominent among early propagators were Dr. Michael Mosley who authored the book *The Fast Diet*. Mosley's documentary *Eat Fast, Live Longer* created a huge upsurge as other nutritionists began to give serious consideration to the idea of intermittent fasting.

Another notable contributor was Kate Harrison. Using her personal experience, she wrote *The 5:2 Diet Book* which made some bold claims such as using the diet method to positively effect anti-aging, Alzheimer, and even cancer. While this is still a subject of scientific research, it is safe to say that using the 5:2 diet method or intermittent fasting method may lead to positive health benefits. (More on the 5:2 intermittent fasting method in subsequent chapters).

Perhaps one of the biggest proponents of modern time intermittent fasting is Dr. Jason Fung. His book *The Obesity Code* was a blockbuster and bestseller as it got a lot of people to consider using intermittent fasting as an effective alternative for other weight loss programs.

In the book, Fung offered great diet suggestions coupled with a detailed series of researches plus his experience as a medical expert to drive home his message: striking a hormonal balance through eating patterns combined with healthy eating may lead to a reversal of weight gain and other health conditions associated with eating habits.

However, the need to seek medical advice for persons who are on some form of medication or have health challenges cannot be over emphasized as sudden disruption to eating patterns may not be well-suited for some individuals. Shortly after Fung and other modern intermittent fasting pioneers' publications, there was a proliferation of personal success stories on the use of intermittent fasting.

Research work is still on-going although most of it tend to highlight the effects in rats. Nevertheless, scientists in Harvard have recently conducted a study that may finally prove the positive effects of intermittent fasting on longevity.

Reports of the Harvard scientific investigations carried out on mitochondrial connections and the effects fasting intermittently has on lifespan was published in *Cell Metabolism* in October 2017. From the study, "*Low-energy conditions such as dietary restriction and intermittent fasting have previously been shown to promote healthy aging. Understanding why this is the case is a crucial step towards being able to harness the benefits therapeutically*" (Harvard T.H. Chan School of Public Health, 2017, n.p.).[3]

The research found that it is possible to increase lifespan through manipulation of the networks of mitochondria in a cell. This manipulation can be done through limitations in diets (fasting) or mimicking such diet limitations using genetics.

Chapter 2: Types of Intermittent Fasting

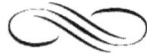

Caution

There are quite a number of intermittent fasting methods that are available. It is important to know which type best suits you in order to practice safe fasting. Before you jump into selecting a type and plunge headlong into this practice, let me give a few pieces of advice.

It is wise to tread carefully when attempting to engage in a practice that may impact on your hormones. Your different hormones are very interconnected, therefore, any major disturbance to one of them may result in an overall destabilization of the others. You really do not want to cause a negative "domino effect" in your system. Your hormones are in charge of regulating your body functions to a very large extent. All such functions as digestion of food, blood pressure regulation, production of energy, and metabolism, etc are intricately regulated by your hormones even if you are not aware that they do. But you will begin to be aware when they stop performing those regulatory functions if you do anything that will interrupt their functions.

Having said all of this, it may appear that intermittent fasting is not as appealing as one may think it is. Well, there is a safe way to do this. I only stated the above because I feel obliged to properly inform my readers of the pros and cons of this practice. Here is a general suggestion for practicing intermittent fasting in a safe way especially for women.

Safe Method for Intermittent Fasting for Women

1. I recommend that you start really slow. Start by adding a few hours to your normal no-eating hours and this time, do not snack in between (else it is no longer intermittent fasting).

2. Let your no-eating time fall between 12 hours to 16 hours. This is ideal and puts less strain on your body especially if you are new to intermittent fasting.

3. If you must fast for longer periods, it is advisable to limit the fast to 24 hours or less at a go. I do not recommend exceeding 24 hours.

4. In your first few weeks (within the first three weeks) it is advisable to avoid fasting on successive days. Allow one- or two-days interval during intermittent fasting. If you decide to fast for 15 hours, for example, you should do so perhaps two or three days spreading the days

throughout the week. Do not carry on the fast for seven consecutive days. Remember, you are just beginning intermittent fasting, so allow your body to gradually get used to it and acclimate your various body systems to it. Continuously fasting for several days in a row in your first few weeks may result in harmful effects.

Intermittent Fasting: Types

Having taken the cautions into proper consideration, let us now turn our attention fully to the different types of intermittent fasting and how they are performed.

5:2

In this type of fasting, you simply eat normally for five days and fast for two days. In those two days of fasting, it is required that you consume only 500 calories per day either by spreading the calories throughout your meals for the day or by consuming it all in one meal (whichever works best for you). So if you choose to use this type of intermittent fasting, you can decide to fast only on Mondays and Tuesdays, for example, limiting your meals for each of these days to only 500 calories. Then from Wednesdays through Sundays, you can resume your normal meals.

This type of intermittent fasting is considered safe for both men and women. It may also be recommended as a good choice for beginners as it does not stop eating even on fasting days (only a restriction on the number of calorie intake). It may as well be the popular choice for easing into fasting since it does not drastically impact your body system in a sudden manner.

There is no fasting window for the 5:2 type of intermittent fasting. All that is required is to limit the total calories to 500 for each of the two days of "fasting" per week. The eating window for the 5:2 fasting method is to simply continue your normal calorie intake for the remaining five days of the week.

Note,however, that there are insufficient scientific studies to back up this type of diet.

16:8

Also called the 8-hour eating window, this type of intermittent fasting involves eating your meals within a period of 8 hours. You should abstain from food (and snacks!) for the rest of the 16 hours of the day. This type of fasting can be done almost daily for the duration you want your intermittent fasting to last. For example, if you choose to do this for the next three months, you could decide to eat all your meals between 12 pm to 8 pm daily (or almost daily) and avoid eating for the rest of the day. What this comes down to is simple: you are skipping breakfast and eating two times (or even three) within 8 hours.

The fasting window for the 16:8 type of intermittent fasting is 16 hours while the eating window is 8 hours (as you probably would have deduced). It is considered safe for both men and women.

Crescendo

This is equally considered as a good way to allow your body to get used to fasting gradually. If you are looking for a method that will not disrupt your hormonal balance, you should consider using this type of intermittent fasting. This involves fasting for a few days in a week for not greater than 16 hours. For example, you could choose to avoid eating for 14 hours on Sundays, Tuesdays, and Thursdays, then eat normally for the rest of the week.

The fasting window for this type of intermittent fasting is usually between 12 to 16 hours. The eating window falls within 8 to 12 hours. And it is considered a safe intermittent fasting method for women.

20:4

In this type of fasting, your meals are all eaten within a period of four hours. For example, you may choose to eat your meals between 3 pm and 7pm every day and avoid food for the rest of the day. So between the hours of 3 pm and 7 pm, you could eat one or two meals and that is all the food you will need for the day. I would recommend you practice this in moderation; that is, do not engage in this for a very long period. A couple of weeks will be considered ideal for you if you are just getting into intermittent fasting.

The fasting window for this type of intermittent fasting is 20 hours, while the eating window is 4 hours only. It is safe for both men and women when done in moderation.

Alternating Days Fasting

Basically, this type of fasting means that you go without food for the whole day and eat freely the following day. In other words, you are eating only half of what you normally would. Water and beverages that contain no calories are allowed on fasting days.

Another version of this type of fasting is to restrict eating to only 500 calories on the days of fasting. The 500 calories can be spread to several meals or consumed at once.

Although this is considered as safe, I would recommend that you perform this type of fasting at most two times a week.

36 Hour Fasting

This type of intermittent fasting involves abstaining from food for the whole day and part of the second day. Here is an example: you commence fasting after you eat dinner on Monday by 8 pm. You then continue fasting for the whole of Tuesday until Wednesday by 8 am before you eat breakfast. Fasting in this way will greatly reduce the urge to overfeed during dinner on the second day.

Although this is a great way to cut down body weight, I would not recommend it for beginners. Women who want to use this method should do their due diligence by consulting their medical experts for advice.

Extended Fasting

This is a type of fasting that continues beyond 48 hours. Yes, it is possible for a person to fast for up to 7 or even 14 days. Our bodies have the capacity to withstand fasting for a very long period although this has to be introduced gradually. If you choose to practice extended fasting, I would strongly recommend that you take a general multivitamin so as not to develop a deficiency for micronutrients. However, do seek medical advice from a qualified physician before taking any multivitamins. Also, I would not recommend anyone (man or woman) to engage in fasting for more than 14 days. This may have a very adverse effect on your health or the general functioning of your hormones.

24 Hour (OMAD) Fasting

Technically, this is considered as the One Meal A Day (OMAD) method because it requires that you eat only once and wait for another 24-hour period before eating again. For example, you may choose to eat lunch at 2 pm and stay away from eating food until the following day by 2 pm before you eat again. In so doing, you are eating every day, but it is limited to only once in a 24-hour period.

The fasting period for this type of intermittent fasting is 24 hours. The eating window is zero hours – all your food is consumed only once after a 24-hour period. This type of fasting is considered safe for men and women provided it is done for not more than two times a week. Moderation is a vital key in this type of fasting.

What to Eat during OMAD Fasting

Although OMAD is pretty simple to understand (and difficult for some beginners to practice), there are a few basic guides to the contents of foods you should eat during the process.

1. *Focus on nutrient-rich foods*: The eating window of OMAD is very limited, and as such you should aim to maximize that period to eat foods that are rich in nutrients and not just bogus calories. Remember that your body needs fats to produce energy, so eat foods that contain healthy fats too.

2. *Maintain your lean muscles*:Your lean muscles need proteins and amino acids to remain in good shape. So be sure to feed your body with enough protein-rich foods.

3. *Carbohydrates are good but not too essential*: There is no backlash for eating fewer

carbohydrates during OMAD fast. With or without carbohydrates, your body will perfume just fine because it will get used to sourcing energy from stored fat. Remember, there is a thing called essential fatty acid, and there is also something known as an amino acid. However, there has never been a mention of any such thing called "essential carbohydrate." (Bernstein, 2018, n.p.).[4]

What to Avoid during OMAD Fasting

Aside from eating junks or unhealthy foods, there are some very healthy foods that may not suit the OMAD fasting. Here's a general guide.

1. *Avoid foods that cause constipation*: avoid foods that are likely to lead to a state of being constipated. Foods such as legumes, beans, cheese, and grains may cause constipation. Fiber is good but should be taken in little quantity.

2. *Avoid foods that are allergenic*: Fasting is likely to heal your gut (if you suffer from gastrointestinal strains); nevertheless, if you consume foods such as legumes and gluten you risk being bloated and this may lead right back to low absorption of necessary nutrients and may also cause some injury to your intestines.

3. *Avoid intake of calorie-rich liquids*: There is a good chance that liquids containing calories may interfere with your digestion process. So keep

away from juices, sodas and all beverages that contain calories. Even too much water during eating may lower the acids in your stomach thereby disrupting the process of absorbing adequate nutrients from your food.

4. *Avoid eating foods that can cause inflammation*:Eating haphazardly is sure to defeat the great anti-inflammatory benefits of fasting. It is advisable to keep away from foods such as hotdogs or grains. To reduce your chances of being foggy the day following your fast, it is best to keep away from candy or ice-cream; although they may not have any negative effect on losing fat, they may cause fogginess.

OMAD Recommended Foods

Let us quickly highlight a couple of recommended foods that you can eat while on OMAD fasting schedule.

1. *Spices (plus herbs too)*: If you are looking for spices and herbs that are known not to contain any calorie, you should consider coriander, parsley, arugula, dill, thyme, etc. These are a great source of micronutrients. Eating maca and reishi are equally good for supporting your body's immune system.

2. *Fats that are healthy*: Olive oil, fish, eggs, avocados, etc. are a great source of healthy fats that can help your hormones. If you are not

allergic to nuts, you can take them in moderation too. Also, consuming raw dairy as well as cheese that is fermented can be a good source of fat too, but don't eat them too much to avoid inflammation.

3. *Carbohydrates*: Rice, turnip, sweet potatoes, beetroots, are but a few examples of whole foods you can take if you choose to increase your carbohydrate intake. It is also fine to eat fruits but not in excess.

4. *Proteins*: Chicken, meat, fish, and eggs, are some good whole foods that can give your body the proteins you need to maintain a good level of amino acid, mineral, and vitamin that will keep you in good health.

5. *Vegetables (healthy ones)*:Vegetables such as spinach and broccoli contain adequate amounts of nutrients you will need. Too much fiber is not advisable, so limit its intake.

Who Should Avoid Intermittent Fasting

The truth is that intermittent fasting is not suitable for every person. It is strongly recommended that you do not attempt intermittent fasting if you fall into the following categories.

•   Those who are suffering from chronic stress

•   If you are known to have eating disorders

which may include anorexia nervosa and bulimia.

- If you have issues with insomnia or sleeping difficulty. All persons having any type of sleep disorders should avoid intermittent fasting.

- If you are lactating or a nursing mother. Breastfeeding your child requires that your body produced extra nutrients to properly feed your child.

- If you are a child under 18 years. Children generally need extra amounts of nutrients to grow properly.

- If you are underweight. Generally, a person whose body weight falls under 18.5 BMI is considered not suitable to practice intermittent fasting.

Those Who Require Supervision to Practice intermittent Fasting

Under certain conditions, you may be able to fast so long as you have adequate medical supervision. However, do remember that the aim of fasting is to keep you in optimal health condition, so if you are already having any of these medical concerns, be sure to have adequate supervision in order not to aggravate your existing medical condition.

- If you are presently taking any prescription

medication. Fasting under these conditions may negatively impact you or disrupt the effect of your medications, hence the need for medical supervision.

- If you are known to suffer from a high amount of uric acid. Also, if you have gouts, you will require medical supervision.

- If you suffer from diabetes mellitus type 1 or type 2 you certainly require supervision to practice intermittent fasting.

Intermittent Fasting for Women: Dos and Don'ts

You could describe this chapter as the "caveat chapter" of this book and you would be correct to some extent. With all the cautions, dos and don'ts, it wouldn't be out of place to feel some sense of caveat, nevertheless, it is a precautionary measure to cause readers to seek proper understanding and guidance before rushing into intermittent fasting in a bid to "keep up with the trend." As with all health-related books, it will be foolhardy to categorically generalize a suggestion as fitting every individual. There truly is no one size fits all, hence the need for all the cautions, dos and don'ts.

So, here are a few more dos and don'ts specifically for women who intend to practice intermittent fasting.

Dos

1. *Check hormone level regularly*: I strongly recommend that women should regularly check their hormonal levels when fasting. On average (and putting it in layman's terms), every 28 days the woman's body repeats a sort of balancing process that is very intricate. If for any reason there is a significant shift in a woman's anxiety level, the frame of mind, type of food, eating habit or pattern, or general state of health, that shift is capable of disrupting her hormones. When this occurs, it may lead to a hormonal imbalance in women – a state no woman would like to remain in as it has the tendency to degenerate into severe health issues in the future. Intermittent fasting has a risk factor of triggering a hormonal imbalance in women if not practiced with moderation or under supervision because of its propensity to induce stress on a woman's body.

Before commencing intermittent fasting, it is important to first check your hormone level. If there are any signs or symptoms of hormonal imbalance, it is best to first tackle that health challenge before commencing your intermittent fasting.

Understand also that the idea that fasting may affect only the woman's sex hormones is not entirely correct. If you have a history of adrenal fatigue, or you have had any health challenge bothering on thyroid disorder, it is very imperative to check your thyroid and cortisol hormones before you begin your intermittent fasting regimen.

2. *Concentrate on high-fat foods*: During intermittent fasting, it is easy for some people to slip into being deficient on calories. To checkmate this, it is recommended that you take foods that are rich in healthy fats. Some nutrient-packed fats are found in foods such as eggs, nut butter, olive oil, coconut oil, and fats that are extracted from healthy animals. Regular intake of these rich fats will ensure that your body has adequate calories and a good supply of nutrients throughout your fasting period. What would be the point in fasting when your body does not have enough nutrients stored up? After all, the purpose of fasting (from the perspective of this book) is to allow your body to use up stored fat.

When you increase the amount of fat in your meals (and of course reduce the carbohydrate), it stabilizes your blood sugar. What happens when you are hungry is that your blood sugar takes a nosedive after some few hours of eating and that causes your body to start to feel hunger. But because you are still fasting even in the face of hunger, your hormones will begin to run rampant because there is no meal to provide sugar (glucose) and that uncomfortable feeling (of no hope of a meal for the next several hours) can lead to stress.

But with the increase in the amount of fat-rich foods, there will be no drop in your blood sugar because your body will no longer depend on glucose from your meals to produce energy. Your body has acclimated to producing energy from fats instead of looking forward to the next sumptuous meal to get its shot of glucose.

3. *Take baby steps*: A gradual shift in your eating pattern is ideally how you should approach intermittent fasting. Jumping straight from eating 3 times a day with regular snacking in between to strictly eating just once in a 24 hour period, might be considered a quantum leap and may not sit well with your body. I would recommend you begin your fasting journey with getting used to rich fat foods even before you commence intermittent fasting. Take a few weeks to get used to that first. Then you can gradually introduce intermittent fasting; perhaps the 16:8 type for about 2 days in a week and watch how your body responds to that. Then you can gradually increase the number of days or the number of fasting hours.

4. *Seek expert advice*: I highly recommend that you consult an expert for advice before embarking on intermittent fasting. Expert guidance would be invaluable to you as it eliminates guesswork and helps you to determine what is best suited to you.

Don'ts

1. *Avoid dieting as much as possible*: Intermittent fasting is not dieting. Its focus is not to sparingly eat calorie-free foods. Intermittent fasting does not target calories as much as it does the amount of time allowed for your body to burn off stored fat or energy. So, during your eating window ensure to eat well not sparingly. Eat nutrient-rich foods and be sure to take your focus off calorie reduction. Intermittent fasting will take care of your calories in a much safer and better way than rigorous dieting ever would.

2. *Avoid intense exercises*: Exercises can be comfortable during fasting, but I strongly recommend that you stay away from rigorous exercises at the early stages of your intermittent fasting. Allow some time for your body to get used to this new pattern of eating before gradually increasing the intensity of your exercises. Understand that you are conditioning your body to adapt to getting energy from a different supply, that is, from majorly relying on glucose to focusing on fats. Do have it in mind that as you are fasting, it is important that your stress level does not suddenly shoot up by any activity you engage in. Stress may probably occur if you engage in strenuous exercises during intermittent fasting and this may cause riots for your hormones.

3. *Avoid weight loss obsession*: Intermittent fasting

may lead to weight loss; true. A lot of people have had success with intermittent fasting with respect to weight loss; very true. Intermittent fasting is an awesome way to get lean muscles, burn body fat, and lose weight; also true. Nevertheless, give yourself a better reason – a higher purpose to go into intermittent fasting. If you obsess about losing weight and begin to coerce your body into losing weight by starving it, you may not get a desirable result. Give yourself other good reasons such as aging gracefully, or sharpening your mind and concentration. There are plenty health benefits derivable from intermittent fasting aside from weight loss. Remember that if you obsess about weight loss, you may inadvertently increase your stress level (by worrying), and that certainly is not good for your hormones.

4. *Avoid forcing yourself*: If it doesn't feel right, halt it. There is no point in compelling yourself to do what does not suit you. The truth is that intermittent fasting is not suitable for everyone, so you will do well to be very attentive to your body as you begin your fasting journey. Any sign of prolonged dizziness or weakness may be signaling you to stop the process. Generally, if the process does not align with who you are, it is probably best to discontinue.

What Next If Intermittent Fasting Is Not Good For You

Okay, so you want to keep in shape and stay

healthy, yet you've determined that intermittent fasting is not good for you, what do you do next? Give up hope and just eat every junk that comes your way and sleep all day? Certainly not!

If intermittent fasting is not good for your body, that is not the end of your health and fitness goal. Simply apply the very basics of essential nutrition which, by the day, is also a necessity even for those who are a good fit for intermittent fasting. Get in the habit of preparing and consuming whole foods. Follow a good workout routine and be committed to it. Additionally, you could find a good coach to help you through the process.

It is quite understandable that you will want to follow the rave of the moment and join "everyone" in doing intermittent fasting, but remember that we are all built differently and some things are just not for everyone. While many men may find this practice easy and natural, it is quite different for a lot of women. So, if you are a woman, it is vital to understudy your body and really find what suits you regardless of what "everyone" seems to be doing. Do have it in mind that there are other ways to stay healthy and keep in shape; so I would recommend that you do not obsess about intermittent fasting to your own detriment.

Chapter 3: Water Fasting: Pros and Cons

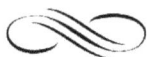

Technically, water fasting is not the same as intermittent fasting. Water fasting is completely going without food and any drink except water throughout the duration of the fast. That is, you fast and when hungry you drink only water, nothing more until your fasting period is over. Typically the fasting period can last for anything from 24 hours to 48 hours or even more. Personally, I would not encourage anyone (man or woman) to fast for longer than 48 hours especially the water fast.

Great care must be taken before attempting water fasting. I definitely would recommend that any woman who intends to practice water fasting should consult an expert. There are many other easier ways to attain and maintain good health and stay fit without necessarily resorting to water fasting. I am not suggesting that water fasting is a no-no for women. I am however stating that it should be approached with a lot of caution.

The Pros

It is possible to lose some weight with water fasting. Since your food intake is completely zero percent, it is very probable that you are going to drop off some weight as your body uses up body fat to keep you up and running.

Water fasting may also lead to a noticeable decline in stress arising from too much oxygen in cells. Too much oxygen in cells can cause cell impairment; a condition known as oxidative stress.

According to Taz Bhatia, M.D., an integrative medicine doctor, "*Oxidative stress is an indication that you are out of balance on a cellular level. This condition can cause excessive fatigue, brain fog, muscle and joint pain, wrinkles and gray hair, poor eyesight, headaches and sensitivity to noise, and a decreased immune system.*" (Bhatia, 2017, n.p.).[5]

Water fasting may reduce this stress thereby causing slow aging. There is also the possibility of a reduction in blood pressure in the individual practicing water fasting.

There is also a likelihood that water fasting can activate autophagy – that is, the elimination of cells that are no longer useful to make way for healthy ones.

The Cons

First of all, it is very obvious that water fasting can leave you really hungry. It is a very strenuous type of fast that may take a serious toll on you; physically draining and mentally exerting you. The stress you may encounter especially for beginners or for prolonged water fasting may not be worth it after all. Have it in mind that too much stress may impact negatively in your hormones (especially the female hormones).

Except you are under close expert monitoring, I do not recommend this type of fast for prolonged hours (beyond 48 hours). It could prove very demanding and may not be suitable for your body at all.

If you are on medication or if you have a history of any disease relating to the liver or kidney, this type of fasting may not be suitable for you. And if you are breastfeeding or you are pregnant, please do not attempt water fasting without strict supervision from qualified medical personnel.

Tips on Water Fasting

The cons may appear to outweigh the pros nevertheless there is a way to go about water fasting in a relatively safe way in other to derive the benefits of the practice. Of course, it goes without saying that before you apply these tips, be sure that you do not have any of the medical conditions stated above and that you do the water fast under supervision especially if you are a woman or if you intend to do it for longer than 48 hours (which I do not recommend).

Here are a few tips to help you with your water fasting:

Brace Up

You are about to embark on an interesting journey that has its ups and downs – it is almost like an adventure. Prepare your mind that you are not going to the hangman, facing a firing squad, or facing a death sentence. It is true that this may appear very challenging but view it from the angle of doing something to improve your overall health and well-being. Equip yourself with sound advice from your medical expert and good books on fasting.

Schedule to Free Time

When you have a tight work schedule or when your family or personal life is full of various activities may not be the best time for performing water fasting. Aim for when you are considerably less burdened with mental and physical activities.

Consider Choosing Short Periods

Limiting the period of your water fast to short periods of about 24 hours is recommended. You can choose to have your water fast maybe just once in an entire week. This is a safer and less strenuous schedule than a prolonged water fasting. And you will still derive the benefits of water fasting from short periods of the fast.

Ease into It

You hear or read about water fasting and the next day you are already fasting. That may be a disaster waiting to happen!Nose-diving into this type of fasting is not recommended at all. Take enough time to prepare yourself. View it as a transition period – from eating food to gradually cutting down your meals, until you eventually stop eating and only take in water for a couple of hours (or for about 2 days. Like I have repeatedly mentioned, I do not recommend water fasting for more than 48 hours except under strict medical supervision). The time it takes to ease into water fasting vary for different individuals. It could be from a couple of weeks to a little above a month, depending on the individual and the recommendation they get from their health experts. The goal is to allow your body to get used to the idea that you intend to take in only water, and you certainly cannot get the body to adjust overnight.

Here's a simple example of how to ease into water fasting over a period of four weeks.

- First Week: Skip breakfast daily. Be consistent about this.

- Second Week: Do not eat breakfast and lunch. Try to keep up with this.

- Third Week: Now reduce your amount of food

for dinner.

- **Fourth Week:** You can now commence water fasting.

Drink Water... Enough Water!

It won't be proper water fast if you don't drink enough water now, would it? Unless otherwise advised by your doctor, the generally recommended amount of water per day for women is about 2.2 liters of water; that is about 9 cups of water. And for men, it is about 3 liters of water or 13 cups of water. (Mayo Clinic, 2017, n.p.). [6]

You know well enough not to drink of all of your water in one go! Space your water intake to span through your day. It is important not to exceed the recommended amount of water because that may lead to some very serious adverse effects on your body. Too much water during fasting may cause a shift in the equilibrium of your body minerals and salt, and this is not what you are aiming for.

Don't Give In to Hunger

You are going to get hungry during water fasting – that is almost a given. I say almost because some veterans may not feel hunger,especially during short (24 hours) water fasting. Nevertheless, when you do get really hungry and your stomach is screaming at you, ride the hunger waves by drinking a cup of water (or two), after which you could simply rest yourself.

Usually, the hunger will subside and eventually fade off. It is also a good practice to get yourself busy in some light activity that will take your mind off the hunger.

Take It Easy With Exercises

If you must work out during water fasting, do ensure to do exercises that are not strenuous or rigorous. Light body movements such as yoga may be great for your body. If yoga feels uncomfortable for you, do something else that is not intense. You could take a walk in nature or whatever appeals to you so long as it is not injurious to your body.

Get Adequate Rest

Rest your body, rest your mind, rest your emotions, and rest your senses. Make sure you give yourself enough rest because water fasting may cause a drain on your resilient energy and staying power. Also, make sure that you get enough sleep and your sleep follows a healthy pattern. Whatever you do, do not weigh down or overwork yourself.If you are not up to it, do not operate machinery or run vehicles. Pay close attention to your body and its messages. When you get a signal to sleep or rest or take a quick nap, by all means listen and do so.

Watch Out for Dizziness

During water fasting, you may have a few occurrences of feeling dizzy especially if you have been in one position for a while and then try to get up suddenly. To avoid this feeling of dizziness, always stand up unhurriedly. You can choose to take in long slow breaths prior to standing up. In the event that you feel dizzy while standing, do promptly lie down gently or simply find a place to sit while you wait for the dizzy feeling to wear off. However, if the dizzy feeling persists or if you begin to lose awareness of your immediate surrounding, I strongly recommend that you discontinue the fasting immediately and consult your doctor promptly.

Gently Break It

When it finally comes to the time to end your water fasting, be extra careful not to rush into feeding your body with too much food too soon. I suggest you start with a juice and give your body some couple of minutes before eating real food. Introduce food gradually; remember that your body has gone without food for a longer period than it is used to, so re-introduce food gently by eating small quantity every few hours.It is a good practice to start with easily digestible foods.

No Junks... Please

Returning to the eating habits that necessitated fasting after you have ended your fast, amounts to a wasted effort. You certainly don't want your body to start accumulating stuff that will make fasting feel like an effort in futility. Fasting alone does not magically transform your health. You need to inculcate good and healthy eating habits as well as regular exercise. Avoid refined sugar and all junk foods.

As earlier mentioned, water fasting may have its own health benefits, but it is very strenuous and may likely trigger stressors especially in women. If you must practice this form of fasting, be sure to visit your health advisor to determine if this is for you.

Chapter 4: Intermittent Fasting: Benefits and Practical Tips

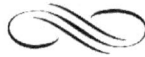

∞

In order to derive any significant benefit from intermittent fasting, first, you must be willing to completely give up snacking at least during the fasting periods. Doing all you can to strictly keep all your meals within the eating window will ensure that you get the best out of intermittent fasting. If you must take in anything, limit it to water or beverages that contain no calories. Remember that the aim is to stay away from food long enough to cause a substantial drop in your insulin levels and for that level to remain that way for a considerable number of hours so that your body will use up a good amount of the energy it has stored. Obviously, this process of burning off stored energy is what makes weight loss one of the widely known benefits of intermittent fasting.

In ancient times people who practiced intermittent fasting for health reasons assumed that they were purifying their body systems (or detoxifying if you will) in order to revivify and cleanse themselves. They were not far from the truth. In more recent times, we have come to realize that intermittent fasting has a good number of benefits, among which are:

Higher Concentration and Brain Power

If humans (and mammals too) are exposed to extreme situations of food scarcity for a long period, the sizes of all but two of their organs will shrink. These two organs are the male testicles and the brain. The testicle retains its size obviously because it is important for producing the next generation.

The brain is chiefly responsible for cognitive functions, and it only makes sense for it to retain its original size and capabilities in order to be able to find food. If for any reason, your brain begins to become extremely foggy, there will be no way to find food and that will definitely result in death. But if anything, in times of starvation the brain becomes more active and alive to seek ways of survival.

Food – too much of it – has a way of dulling our mental sharpness. Think back to the times when you were completely satiated, what comes to you naturally:a drive to focus and get things done or a desire to just sleep for a while and even lazy around for a bit? Obviously, a satiated feeling squelches your drive to put your brain to work; it dulls your brain. Hunger tends to quicken your cognitive abilities and too much food is likely to impede your mental keenness.

There is no scientific study to support the idea that intermittent fasting has any harmful effect on mental alacrity. Fasting does not negatively impact attention, moods, sleep, reaction time, or any cognitive functions. On the contrary, mental functions seem to be boosted during fasting.

Possible Inhibition of Alzheimer's Disease

In simple terms, Alzheimer's disease has been closely linked to obesity. Gaining weight during one's middle age may increase the chances of Alzheimer's disease. Equally, the accumulation of abnormal proteins has been found to indicate Alzheimer's disease.

"It is believed that these abnormal proteins destroy the synaptic connections in the memory and cognition areas of the brain" (Fung, 2016, n.p.). [7]

Fasting can lead to a reduction in weight gain as well as stimulate the removal of abnormal proteins from the body. In other words, it is possible for intermittent fasting to have a significant positive effect on obesity and accumulation of abnormal proteins; both of which have been suggested to have a link to Alzheimer's disease.

Weight Loss

When you eat fewer calories or you burn a good amount of calories continually, you are definitely on a path that is likely to result in weight loss.

These two – eating fewer calories and burning calories – are both incidental to intermitted fasting. However, counting calories is not a requirement for intermittent fasting, nevertheless, if you do not eat too much during your eating hours (to compensate for lack of eating during the fasting period), you are most likely to take in fewer calories than you normally would if you were not doing intermittent fasting.

In 2014, a review study indicated that intermittent fasting can result in considerable loss of weight. The review study shows that within a three to twenty-four-week period, three to eight percent of body weight was reduced due to intermittent fasting. (Science Direct, 2014, p. 302-311).[8]

Possible Activation of Cellular Cleansing

Our body cells are programmed to die off after a number of cell-divisions. This allows for new cells that are more healthy and active to replace them. This process may be loosely referred to as cellular cleansing; getting rid of worn out cells to make way for the new.

Generally, when we eat, insulin levels increases and when we fast, the opposite happens; insulin levels decrease. But fasting or not eating does not just trigger a decrease in insulin levels but triggers an increase in glucagon – the hormone (in the pancreas) that raises blood sugar level. Glucagon has an opposite function to insulin. So, when we fast, our glucagon level increases and this leads to clearing of worn out cells. This process is fully discussed in a subsequent chapter about autophagy.

Possible Positive Effect on Aging

If you have a mostly inactive lifestyle and are above age 30, there is a high chance that your growth hormones are gradually falling into deficit phase. Our bodies produce adequate amounts of growth hormones when we are much younger.However, as we age, there is a gradual decline in the growth hormones which eventually culminates in a noticeable decrease in lean body mass and a buildup of fat in the body. This fat is usually noticeable in the abdomen area. Equally, as we age, there is a decrease in our body's bone mineral density. This downturn in our growth hormone as we age can make us begin to feel older and even look it too.

Fasting is known to burn stored fats and beyond that, it can also help to keep our lean muscles intact. Fasting can lead to the production of substantial amounts of growth hormones that can allow our bodies to age gracefully.

Generally, when we fast, we give our growth hormones a boost. And our growth hormones may have the following positive effects on our bodies:

- It can significantly cut down evidence of aging, in other words, you grow older looking younger than your age.

- It can greatly reduce the accumulation of fat in our body.

- Growth hormones can reinforce our bones

- In order to support the repair of damaged muscles, growth hormones can increase the production of fresh protein tissues.

- It can help to keep our body organs in prime conditions even as we age

- It can help to maintain a lean body

- Growth hormones support optimal nail and hair growth

Others Benefits of Intermittent Fasting

Other benefits may also include:

- Promoting or boosting energy

- There is significant muscle mass increase, that is to say, an increase in your lean muscle

- Reduction in sugar level and blood insulin

- Reduction in cravings for sugar

- Possible Reversal of type 2 diabetes

- Improvement in sleep pattern

- Significant improvement in the burning of fat

- Reduction of cholesterol

- Reduction in bloating

- Decreased inflammation

- Noticeable improvement in digestion

- There is a noticeable increase in the resistance that your body can put up against diseases as a direct result of an increase in the rate of the cell stress response.

- And there is *"a reduction in oxidative stress and inflammation and Improvement around insulin sensitivity in overweight women"* (Kettle and Fire, 2018, n.p.).[9]

On a general note, if you approach intermittent fasting in an attitude of detoxifying your body, you will enjoy its several benefits. Allow your body to "eat" its own food or feed itself, and when you do (through fasting), your body and its intelligent cells will work their "magic" to rid your system of broken cells and free radicals.

Practical Tips for Fasting

Like every other thing in life, fasting requires some real-world, hands-on considerations and quite a bit of practice in order to become good at it. Here are some awesome tips that are very likely to help you. You will be correct to a large extent if you view them as this book's "FAQ" section on intermittent fasting. Remember, if you allow your body to get used to this process, you open yourself up to enjoy the freedom from constantly thinking about eating.

Dear Woman, Find a Good Reason to Fast

Do not fast simply because you want your body fat to go from 20% to 13% for example. That's not a good enough reason to fast. Perhaps what you should consider is dieting. Do not fast because you want to keep your pregnancy weight in check. That may be very unwise for you and your unborn baby. Do not fast because you are seeking to get a boost for your regular fitness sessions.

If you must fast let it be for cogent reasons such as your neurologist recommending it to help reverse the effects dementia; an oncologist suggesting the use of fasting to boost the results of chemotherapy; you have a large amount of fat that really requires losing.

Aim for Results, not Plaques

First of all, your fasting goals shouldn't be a subject for public consumption. So understand that no one is actually taking scores except you (and those who are genuinely interested in supporting your goals). For this reason, there is no point trying to impress anyone by going for the longest fast possible. You are a woman first and foremost, so allow your body some quality time to rest from the stress of fasting. Even though overcoming hunger and nasty headaches as you coerce your body to pull through a difficult fasting regimen may earn you a pat on the shoulder, consider what the negative impact will be on your hormones in the long run.

A Gentle Break-Fast

Fasting window is over! Finally, it's time to eat and you rush to munch a mouthful of your favorite meal devouring as much as you can in the shortest possible time to make up for missed meals. Newsflash: you are going to hurt your stomach with that attitude. Slow down! The tendency to rush into consuming foods in large quantity can be tamed if you take on the right attitude, and that would be to gently break your fast.

Hurling down large amounts of food into your stomach immediately after fasting may lead to some very unpleasant stomach distress. Whatever food you choose to use in breaking your fast, be sure to make it light and in small quantity at first and wait for some minutes before eating a full meal. For example, you can choose to break your fast with some veggies, and then wait for about 20 minutes for your body to get used to eating again after going a long time without food. This waiting period is likely to make hunger waves subside after which you can eat your normal meal.

Handling Hunger During Fasting

The worry about hunger probably tops the list of concerns about fasting. For people who are new to the idea of fasting, the fear of hunger may be the number one reason they are reluctant to start the process.

However, hunger has a way of passing or wearing off if you distract yourself by getting busy. Remember that your body is accustomed to getting its energy supply from the meals you eat, but fasting makes your body gradually turn to stored fat for its energy supply. So at first, you may experience bouts of hunger. Do not fret. It will pass with time and when your body begins to adapt to sourcing for energy from stored fat, you will hardly feel hungry during fasting.

I would recommend that you get yourself busy at work, at home or in any activity that will keep your focus away from food, eating, fasting hours, or how slowly time is passing.

Liquids to Take During Intermittent Fasting

Please note that different types of fasting have different requirements. Some types of fasting require complete abstinence from all foods and liquids including water. Others forbid eating of meat during fasting. In this type of intermittent fasting, taking of liquids is ideal and highly recommended in order not to be dehydrated.

Taking liquids or beverages may also help in suppressing hunger during fasting periods. However, keep in mind that beverages or liquids containing calories are a no-no.Here are some nice liquids I would recommend to take during intermittent fasting.

1. *Water*: It is a good practice to stay well-hydrated throughout your fasting period. It is advisable to drink about two liters of clean water throughout the duration of your fasting as well as when you are not fasting, that is, for the entire day. You can drink enough water in the mornings to make sure that your body gets sufficient water to kick-start the day. You can choose to add natural flavors like lime or lemon to your water, but whatever you do, make certain to keep away from sweeteners and artificial flavors.

2. *Broth*: Broths are excellent for fasting periods. You can choose a mixed vegetable broth or a bone broth, both are great choices. However, be wary of buying broths inside of cans. Take the time to prepare (or get someone to help you prepare) your broth at home.

3. *Coffee*: There is a great chance for the caffeine present in coffee to lead to an increase in your body metabolism. This is good for burning of fat. Decaffeinated and caffeinated coffees are both good for fasting periods. Whatever you add to your coffee (for example, cinnamon) be sure it

does not contain calories and the flavors are not the artificial types.

4. *Tea*: Teas are also a good choice of beverage to take during fasting. You can also choose to spice up your tea with nutmegs but the artificial flavor rule also applies here. All types of teas are great, but green tea has an extra dose of antioxidants which may help to promote metabolism. This, perhaps, accounts for why dieticians recommend green tea as it may help in significant weight loss.

5. *Cinnamon*: Technically, cinnamon is not liquid or a beverage, but it is a great addition to beverages. Aside from its likelihood to suppress the feeling of hunger, cinnamon may equally lead to the lowering of sugar in the blood. Add a nice amount of ground cinnamon to your beverages to give it a great taste and also enjoy its health benefits.

6. *Chia seed*: Rich in omega 3 fatty acids, Chia seeds can be taken in their dry form or soaked in water to form a thick pudding. It is believed that Chia seeds may help to reduce appetite during fasting.

Give It About a Month

For you to accurately determine if intermittent fasting suits you, you need to give it time, perhaps about a month or at least 3 weeks. Unless you are under any medication or have an ongoing health issue (in which case you need to seek medical advice before going into fasting), you should give your body adequate time to get used to this pattern of eating and show you whether to continue or put an end to it. However, if during the first few days you notice very uncomfortable and prolonged dizziness, it is advisable to discontinue the process immediately and promptly seek medical advice.

Flexibility

You have the freedom of mapping out a fasting program that fits into your lifestyle and schedules. Let intermittent fasting fit into your schedules rather than feeling you are being boxed into something that doesn't suit your lifestyle. It is your life; others (well-meaning people by the way) can only suggest what you should do, but ultimately, you should allow room for flexibility. Do not strictly follow unrealistic schedules as if they are carved in stone; adjust them to suit you.

Perform More Tasks in the Mornings

Most fasting windows are usually scheduled to skip breakfast. Use your morning hours to get your best work done. You will find you are very productive during fasting especially when you wake up early. Adjust your productive tasks to fit into your morning schedules.

Get Active

There is no reason to just sit and spend the whole day lying around the house because you are fasting. Go out. Take a walk. Visit someone. Do chores. Workout. Just do something – anything to get active so that your body can really use up that stored fat.

Your First Meal of the Day is Important

By"first meal," I do not necessarily mean breakfast. I mean the meal you take to break your fast. When you break your fast ensure that you eat healthy because it has a way of carving the path which you are likely to take for the rest of your meals.

Follow a Structure, Then Play Around Later

It is important to find a good intermittent fasting program and follow it diligently for at least a month. This has two main benefits. First of all, it allows you to know if intermittent fasting is for you; and secondly, it allows you to learn the ropes – to get a good handle on how intermittent fasting works.

After you have determined that intermittent fasting is for you by following a good structure for about a month, you can then begin to play with it. Yes, play with it – try different methods that appear appealing to find which sits well with you. For example you may want to use the 16:8 intermittent fasting, so you eat three meals in a day with the first meal at 1 pm, the second at 5 pm, and the third at 9 pm and then you commence fasting for the next 16 hours breaking it at 1 pm the following day.

You could choose to joggle the timing of eating a bit to 11 am, 3 pm, and 7pm. And you can also choose to eat only twice so you adjust your time of eating to whatever time suits you before fasting for the rest of the 16 hours.

Eat Healthy Foods

There is no point fasting for 2 days, keeping your calories to 500 max, and then follow it with 5 days of eating junk! For God's sake that's just counterproductive. Resist the temptation to stuff your body with foods you know are not good for you. Stick to eating whole foods and vegetables.

Keep It to Yourself

It is important to keep your decision to start fasting for yourself especially if you are new to it. Although there is some buzz about intermittent fasting, there are a lot of people who are yet to really get the grasp of it. .. These category of people will do all in their capacity to discourage you. Remember that every individual is unique. What may not work for someone may work well for another. So keep it to yourself until you are surefooted.

Chapter 5: Different Women, Different Results

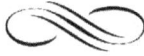

The Female

D ifferent women react differently to even something as commonly shared among all women as the menstrual cycle. In fact, even in a particular individual female, she may react one way in one cycle and react another way in another cycle. This also applies to intermittent fasting and fasting in general. There is no one size fits all when it comes to the woman's body and her reactions.

This should, however, not be viewed as a "curse" or a disadvantage of some sort, neither should it be seen as some form of unfairness to the female gender. Rather,it should be viewed somewhat as a highly evolved way for the woman's body to signal her of what is good and not good for her at every given moment. These signals come very early to warn (or encourage) a pattern that has been noticed in the female body. This happens because of the delicateness of the female body; a body designed to reproduce young ones to carry on the perpetuation of the human species.

For optimal body performance, the hormones in your body need to be at equilibrium (or near perfect balance) at all times. The slightest change in eating habit, stress level, or psychological and physiological distress may lead to a significant hormonal imbalance in your body. This is why it is important to know exactly what works for you as an individual woman. You should not risk any damage to your hormones in a bid to get the "good" health and fitness results of another person even if the person is a woman like you.

What Fasting Does to The Female Hormone

Fasting is a good lifestyle. Many have argued that it is the normal way humans are designed to live: eat and go without food until you have used up what you ate before eating another meal. Eating three to six meals in a day may not allow your body to properly use up the energy (sugar and other nutrients) you are supplying to it. It is like stuffing your body with excess energy when it has not consumed close to half of what it has before. This may lead to excess fat stored in your body and can cause too much weight. Too much weight is associated with insulin resistance, diabetes, and other diseases.

Fasting can help the body to burn up enough amounts of energy before taking in new food. But what does it do to the hormones? What effects does it have especially on the female hormones? Remember that hormones are like the messengers or communication agents of the body; sending and receiving signals all the time. When a woman goes without food for a long time (fasting), there is a higher tendency for her hormones to go out of order. Chiefly among these hormones are insulin, cortisol, progesterone, and estrogen. Some women may experience irregular menstrual cycles, or a complete stoppage of their monthly flow when they experiment with intermittent fasting.

Let us take a quick look at some hormones in the female that might be impacted during intermittent fasting.

Progesterone and Estrogen

For a woman to get pregnant and for her to remain in a general state of well-being, it is important that her hypothalamic-pituitary-gonadal (HPG) remains in a healthy state. And just in case you are wondering what HPG is, it is the means of communication between your brain and your ovaries. When the communication channels are in good order, your ovaries receive signals from your brain (at the right time) and then releases progesterone and estrogen.

Fasting seems to impact women more because of their higher level of kisspeptin which scientists have suggested causes sensitivity to stress-producing activities like fasting (I shall explain what kisspeptin is in a moment). This sensitivity caused by kisspeptin can make the hormones in a woman's body go completely out of balance and may lead to things like an irregular menstrual cycle. There is also a possibility of the hormonal imbalance to negatively impact a woman's fertility and even her metabolism.

The above notwithstanding, it important to always keep in mind that no two women (and as a matter of fact, no two humans) are the same. Some women may actually find intermittent fasting as a tool that greatly improves their overall well-being, while others may not have the same experience.

Cortisol

Cortisol is the stress hormone. When you are under stress, your adrenal gland produces the hormone cortisol. However, fasting in some women interferes with this function. It either keeps the cortisol level high when it ought to be low, or it keeps it low when it ought to be high. Sometimes it can keep the cortisol level continually high or continually low. A woman that has this type of issue may not be the best fit for intermittent fasting.

Thyroid

The effects of your thyroid hormones are felt in every part of your body and in every living cell in your body. What this means is that, if your thyroid hormones are out of whack, you can be sure your health is also out of whack. Intermittent fasting is just one out of the many reasons your thyroid hormones can go out of balance. So if you suspect an issue with your thyroid hormone, it is best to see a medical expert to determine if it is caused by intermittent fasting or other issues.

But Why Should Female Reproductive Hormones Take More Hit Than Men's?

Before I go into a little bit of the science about the possible reason, let us ask a few more logical questions, perhaps in answering them, we may find the answer to the earlier question.

Are you capable of reproducing your kind? Are you capable of reproducing a healthy offspring of your species that will thrive and also continue the lineage? Now, it takes a mammal with a womb to be able to do this. And that mammal with a womb needs additional nutrients in her body to prepare the womb for her expected young. And because that mammal is also specially designed to reproduce, her body is very sensitive to the slightest change in her eating habit. That mammal is the delicately built female human.

Now, let's add a teeny-weeny bit of science to that. Changes in eating habits and patterns are more likely to affect the woman than the man. Why this is so is not absolutely certain; however, it may be linked to a molecule used in passing information between neurons. This molecule (which is more or less protein) is called kisspeptin; it functions to promote the production of hormones like progesterone and estrogen that are responsible for ovulation in women and production of testosterone in men for reproduction. These hormones are interconnected to other hormones in the body and are sensitive to the hormones that are in charge of controlling the feeling of satiation and the feeling of hunger (ghrelin, insulin, and leptin are linked to this feelings).

The level of kisspeptin in women is higher than that of men. What this means is that their hormones are more alive to slight changes in the overall balance of body energy. Perhaps this is why when women fast, it is likely to lead to a sharp decline in their kisspeptin levels which in turn may affect their hormones for reproduction.

There is no scientific study to show the effect of fasting on human female reproductive hormones; however, there is evidence of such studies on rats. And until such a time when there will be one, we can only make do with what is available and tread carefully since this is an uncertain area of study. Remember, there are no 100% guarantees.

Perhaps a quick look at one study to buttress the above will be a great idea at this point.

One of such study was published in a research

article in January 2013 and titled *"Intermittent Fasting Dietary Restriction Regimen Negatively Influences Reproduction in Young Rats: A Study of Hypothalamo-Hypophysial-Gonadal Axis"* (Kumar and Kaur, 2013, n.p.). [10]

The study adopted the following method.

A total of 20 regular-sized rats (10 for each of the sexes) were the subjects. The rats were divided into two groups, and for a period of 12 weeks, one group was allowed to eat any time they felt like eating. For the other group, they were allowed access to food on alternating days effectively making the rats to fast.

At the end of the observation period, there was a 19 percent loss in body weight recorded among the female rats that took part in the fasting. There was a noticeable reduction in the sizes of their ovaries, and also a reduction in the level of their glucose.Leptin levels in the female rats that fasted were far much lower than those who fed daily. Production of kisspeptin was significantly down too.

Generally, the study shows that the hormones of the female rats were more negatively impacted by the experiment than their male counterparts. Both hormones in charge of appetite and reproduction were negatively impacted in the female rats which were made to take part in the fasting.

The question that is begging for an answer now is: what is the implication of this for us humans? Should all women avoid intermittent fasting and indeed any fasting all in all?

I will like to point out that it is not quite easy to put in black and white what this means for female humans, and with mixed reports from anecdotes of many women who have practiced intermittent fasting. However, it would be safe to proceed with caution in the understanding that each woman is different, and her body reacts very differently from any other woman (and female rats too!)

Energy Balance

It is important to note that it is not only the female reproduction that may take a hit from a hormonal imbalance that may occur due to fasting. So even if you are no longer interested in getting pregnant, you should be aware that when something makes your body's reproductive hormones go out of whack, there is more to the story.

Aside from fasting, there are quite a number of physical and mental activities that are capable of disrupting the energy balance of a woman and which may likely affect her hormonal balance. Not every hormonal imbalance in women are caused by a change is eating habit. Here are some other stressors that may lead to hormonal or energy imbalance in women:

- Long-lasting inflammations, infections, or illnesses

- Some prescription medication

- Excessive strain in your body in the form of excessive physical exercises

- Inadequate recovery time from workouts or lack of enough rest

- Continuously eating very small amounts of food

- Involving in poor nutritional habits

- Excessive mental stress (worrying, anxiety, fear, etc)

It is also quite possible that a woman may already have an ongoing issue with some of these physical and mental activities which may not be apparent.However, when fasting is introduced into the mix, it may exaggerate and bring to fore the effects of these underlying stressors. The woman who may not have been paying attention to her body would simply conclude that fasting has caused her current health predicament.

A negative energy balance can result from a mix of any of these stressors, and may ultimately put a halt to a woman's ovulation. But why should psychological stress (alone or in combination with any other stressor) result in a hormonal imbalance in women? Well, first of all, it is not only peculiar to women to have a negative effect on hormones due to psychological stress. It has a common undesirable effect in both men and women. Furthermore, the human mind (and by extension, the body) does not have the capability to distinguish between a real-life situation and an imagined situation. Our bodies react in a similar fashion to things happening in physical reality and things happening in our imagination; as long as we feel them, the mind and body assume they are real. (Have you wondered why your body reacts physically to a dream or nightmare?)

The Role of Our Perceptions

Putting all of these pieces together; hormones, energy balance, and stressors, it would be fairly correct to say that a woman may react negatively to intermittent fasting if her body perceives fasting as a major stressor.This may eventually lead to negative effects on her reproductive health. And as a matter of fact, anything that is capable of affecting a woman's reproduction negatively is more than likely to have an undesirable effect on her overall health.

We are not rats. Humans are capable of generating and controlling their own thoughts and perceptions as well as controlling their feelings. And although we may not be able to accurately generalize and place a finger squarely on the power of mind over matter (as scientific studies would require), we also cannot dismiss or deny the significant role our states of mind play in our overall health. I mean, considering the placebo effect, we truly must acknowledge, to a certain degree, the power of our perceptions.

Having said all of that, it is very important to be pragmatic and empirical when dealing with the workings of our bodies. Intermittent fasting should not be done based on some anecdotal account from a motivational speaker. It is quite useful if you would pay attention to what your body tells you.

A Woman's Body Tells Her When Not to Fast

Since there are lots of gray areas and so much uncertainty around the issue of women fasting, I would generally recommend that women should approach intermittent fasting with a touch of conservativeness. A woman that wants to have a shot at intermittent fasting should begin with a gentle regimen and be ever alert to what her body is telling her.

A woman should discontinue intermittent fasting when any of the followings occur:

- If you observe any irregularity in your menstrual cycle or if it completely stops

- If you notice frequent mood swings

- If there is a significant drop in your ability to be tolerant to stress

- If you begin to notice the appearance of acne or you begin to have a dry skin

- If you observe that it takes too much time before you can fully recover from exercises

- If you notice that your hair starts to fall off

- If you notice that you easily catch common bugs or you notice that it takes a longer time for your injuries to heal

- If you observe a decline in your interest in romance or you notice that sex becomes a chore that you'd rather avoid

- If you start having issues with insomnia or you tend to be deprived of sleep (finding it difficult to fall asleep or sleep well)

- If you notice that you are cold most of the time

- If you notice a significant drop in the time it takes for your food to digest

- If you observe a continuous irregular beating of your heart

Insulin Resistance: What It Is

Under normal circumstances, the hormone called insulin sends signals to our cells to extract glucose from our blood. This signal is received by the cells and acted upon. However, when the cells in some organs such as the liver or in body fat and muscles begin to disregard this signal, we say there is a resistance to insulin. Our body is primarily fueled by glucose – or blood sugar. So when your body cells develop a resistance to insulin, in effect, it is rejecting or resisting the necessary fuel it needs to keep you functioning well.

Insulin Resistance: Causes

Age may be a factor for insulin resistance; so is genetics and possibly ethnicity too. But the main culprits behind the rejection of the insulin signal are:

- Excess fat (especially in the belly region)

- Overweight (obesity)

- Smoking

- Improper sleeping habit or sleep deprivation

- Not exercising (being inactive)

Your body puts up a good fight as it tries to overcome insulin resistance by producing more insulin. But this fight cannot go on forever. Sooner or later, your pancreas cells get tired from the constant production of more insulin, and they give up. With time, your glucose level (or sugar level in the blood) may begin to increase which may, in turn, lead to prediabetes or type 2 diabetes. Another disease that you may be prone to is the

NAFLD – Non-Alcoholic Fatty Liver Disease. NAFLD increases your chances of heart diseases and liver damage. (American Journal of Managed Care, 2013, n.p.).[11]

Insulin Resistance: Signs and Symptoms

1. *Too much fat around the waist*: a good way to know if you are tending towards having insulin resistance is to simply take a good look at your waist or abdomen area. Too much fat around there may be an indication that you run the risk of developing insulin resistance.

2. *Signs of metabolic syndrome*: metabolic syndrome increases the chances of having insulin resistance. Having any three or more of the symptoms listed below may be a sign of metabolic syndrome.

   - High blood pressure

   - High blood sugar

   - High fasting blood sugar

   - High triglycerides

   - Low high-density lipoprotein levels (HDLs)

3. *Dark patches on the skin*: in serious cases of insulin resistance, dark patches may begin to appear on your skin. This condition is referred to as acanthosis nigricans. Often times this dark

patches will appear on the armpit or behind the neck. And in some cases, it may also appear on the groin. There seems to be no cure (for now) for this condition. (Rowland, 2017, n.p.).[12]

Insulin Resistance:Prevention

There are several ways to prevent (or reverse) insulin resistance. Some of the more common ways are:

1. *Weight loss*: any good weight loss program (such as keto dieting) can improve your chances of preventing insulin resistance. Losing "*even just 7 percent of your body weight can lower your risk of developing diabetes.*" (Rowland, 2017, n.p.). [12] Intermittent fasting has one of its very obvious benefits as weight loss. It is a good practice if you can fast intermittently to help prevent insulin resistance.

2. *Exercise regularly*: hitting the gym for at least 30 minutes of workout will greatly improve your chances of preventing insulin resistance. If you are combining intermittent fasting with some exercises, do remember to keep it low-impact.

3. *Get adequate sleep*: give your body enough rest at night. You need it to keep stress at bay and stall any chances of an increase in blood sugar level. One night of poor sleep, researchers found, is almost equivalent to insulin resistance caused by six months of consuming foods that are rich in

fat! (Broussard, 2015, n.p.).[13]

Chapter 6: Intermittent Fasting: Myth vs. Reality

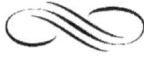

A s with any subject that has not been fully understood, there are a lot of myths about intermittent fasting. Too many people have become "overnight experts" on fasting and are eager to dish out their pieces of advice to anyone who cares to listen. Some of these myths are deeply rooted in fear while others are just sheer ignorance. Let us take a look at some myths about intermittent fasting.

Fasting Triggers "Starvation Mode"

There is this common claim that intermittent fasting or fasting, in general, will activate "starvation mode" in your body. What that means is that your body senses that you are starving, so it tries to conserve energy by significantly reducing the amount of fat it burns. While this explanation is very correct, it does not hold true for short periods of fasting. On the contrary, intermittent fasting can increase metabolic activities which lead to the burning of fat. The only time your body goes into starvation mode while fasting is when you engage in prolonged fasting periods.

Intermittent Fasting is Harmful to Health

This myth seems to stem from complete ignorance of how the body works. There are no two individuals that are exactly the same. So we cannot assume that because one person experienced adverse effects on their health during fasting, therefore every other person is liable to have the same effect. There are a number of reasons fasting may not be good for a particular individual, but that does not necessarily translate into a general issue. The truth is, intermittent fasting or fasting for short periods is safe and has numerous health benefits. However, the practice may not be suitable for everyone.

You Lose Muscles When You Fast

Some people hold the belief that intermittent fasting can make you lose your muscle. However, studies have shown that we actually can retain better muscle mass when we fast. (US National Library of Medicine, 2011, n.p.). [14]There exists no shred of evidence to support the claim that we lose muscles more during fasting than during dietary practices that restrict calories.

Frequent Eating Reduces Hunger

This is a subject that has mixed evidence. Some studies suggest that frequent eating or snacking can reduce hunger in some people, while other studies suggest that it can increase hunger in some people. Yet other studies have shown that it has no effect at all. (US National Library of Medicine, 2013, n.p.).[15]This boils down to individual differences. To some people, snacking in between meals or eating frequently helps to reduce hunger in them nevertheless, that does not apply everyone.

You Get Fat If You Don't Eat Breakfast

There is simply nothing spectacular or magical about breakfast especially in connection to gaining weight. Randomized controlled trial does not put forth any concrete evidence to support the theory of gaining weight by skipping breakfast. Rather it simply shows that there is no difference in weight gain or loss when one skips breakfast or eats breakfast. This too is a subject of individual difference.

You Must Lose Weight During Intermittent Fasting

This is a common misconception. Intermittent fasting does not always guarantee that you will lose weight. Except done properly, intermittent fasting may prove ineffective. If you go about eating everything that comes your way during your eating window, the chances of losing weight are very slim or even nonexistent. Also, if you continue to cheat during the fasting window, there is no guarantee that you will lose weight.

Eat As Much As You Wish After Fasting

You are likely to sabotage all the efforts you put

into intermittent fasting if you eat large amounts of food after your fasting. You should continue to eat your normal sized meals after you have ended your fast. Doing otherwise may not produce the desired effect you wish to get from intermittent fasting. What will be the point of fasting all day only to end your fast and eat a meal that has the combined size of all the day's meal put together? You simply shoot yourself in the foot.

It Is Harmful to Exercise During Fasting

Not only is it safe to exercise during fasting, but it also helps your body to burn fat that has already been stored instead of trying to burn calories that are newly ingested from your meals. This is why it is a good practice to exercise in the morning on an empty stomach.

The Results from Intermittent Fasting Are the Same for Everyone

This is completely bogus and far removed from the truth. First of all, intermittent fasting is not even of one type. Different people practice different forms of intermittent fasting, and their results vary depending on what type of intermittent fasting they choose to practice and their body differences. As earlier mentioned, no two individuals are exactly the same. There are a lot of indices that can lead to different results for different people even when they practice the same type of intermittent fasting. It is advisable to find what type of intermittent fasting works best for you and focus on it. Your result may or may not be the same as the next person's and, in fact, results are not typical.

Intermittent Fasting Makes You Fit and Very Healthy

By itself, intermittent fasting is not an automatic ticket to leanness and great health. There is a need to combine fasting with quality exercise and healthy eating and living for it to result in great health and a fit body.

Metabolism Slows Down During Fasting

There is a huge difference between limiting the amount of calorie you take in and controlling the time that you take in calories. The focus of intermittent fasting is mainly on the latter. There is no evidence to show any change to your metabolic rate when you delay your meal for some few hours. It is only whenyoubegin to starve – that is when you start to under-eat – that changes begin to take place in your metabolic rate. However, intermittent fasting is not the same as under-eating.

Intermittent Fasting Leads to Too Much Eating

Some people have the belief that fasting can lead to too much eating during the eating window to make up for the meals missed (or supposedly lost calories) during fasting. While it is true that some people have the tendency to eat a lot after they break their fast, it does not hold true in all cases. When done properly, intermittent fasting has a way of suppressing hunger (taking of liquids in between), and with time cravings seem to pass, and the feeling of hunger and subsequent desire to "compensate" or make up for meals lost will fade. Intermittent fasting may even lead to a reduction in the overall amount of food the individual consumes as the body adapts to getting its food from another source rather than from meals consumed.

Chapter 7: Intermittent Fasting and Keto Diet

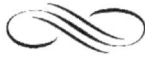

Keto Diet: What It Is

The term "keto" derives from ketones which are produced from the breakdown of fat. Ketones are substitute sources of energy to the body when the main source (glucose) is not readily available.

A keto diet is a specially designed regimen that makes your meals consists of very low carbohydrate and high fat targeted at making you effectively burn more fat. Keto diet has gainedsomewhatcelebrated fame in the world of dieting and nutrition because of its obvious weight loss benefit and other not too obvious health benefits.

The keto diet is aimed at getting your body to breakdown fat to produce an alternative source of fuel for your body. And this alternative source (ketones) is produced faster when you stop eating or when you fast. But then can we stop eating forever? Certainly, no one would even want to attempt that. This is where the keto diet comes into play. You could eat a keto diet forever and still produce enough alternative source of fuel for your body.

Avoid It If...

Keto diet is considered safe for many people, however, for some reasons, it may not be suitable for everyone. If you fall into any of the following categories, it is best to avoid a keto diet or consult your doctor before proceeding.

- If you are pregnant

- If you are breastfeeding

- If you are taking medications for your blood pressure

- If you are treating diabetes

The Relationship between Intermittent Fasting and Keto

For a clearer understanding of the relationship between intermittent fasting and keto, let us take a quick look at what ketosis is?

Ketosis

In simple terms, ketosis is the activity that causes the use of ketone bodies as a source of energy to sustain the body. It is a metabolic process that breaks down fat released into your bloodstream and then converted into energy molecules that are used as a primary source of fuel for the body. These molecules are called ketone and are produced in the liver.

Your brain is obviously a powerful organ that requires a lot of energy to power it. And although your body can run on fat, your brain can't do that, at least, not directly. Your brain is powered by energy supply from glucose alone... well, not glucose alone; glucose and ketone. So, even though fat may not provide direct energy to your brain, it does so when converted into ketone.

When you eat your normal meals that are high in carbohydrates, your body converts the carbohydrate into its fuel (glucose). Excess glucose extracted from your meals are then stored in form of glycogen. Now when you stop eating food, or you perform exercises, the glucose in your body is used up quickly and your body turns to the glycogen it stored earlier and begins to use it as fuel.This also happens when you start eating foods that are low in carbohydrate (keto dieting). If you do not supply glucose to your body on time (as in fasting), the supply of glycogen is eventually exhausted, and your body is forced to shift its attention to another source of energy – fat.

Keto dieting (or ketogenic diet) is specially designed to compel your body to source for energy from ketone bodies which are produced from the breakdown of fat stored in your body. Fat (ketone bodies) is a more stable source of energy than carbohydrate (glucose) which comes from your meals.

The Link

What then is the link between intermittent fasting and keto?

Basically, intermittent fasting limits your food intake to a shorter period for the whole day (8, 4, or even 0-hour eating window) and makes you go without food for longer periods (12, 16, 20, or even 24 hours fasting window). That means your food intake (and as a side bonus, your calorie intake) is lower.

We have earlier explained that your body stores glycogen (excess glucose) and continues to use them as a source of energy to power you. When glycogen is exhausted, your body turns to fat for energy supply.

Here then is the link: intermittent fasting already has the effect of burning off glycogen, so it will boost the speed with which you get into ketosis by helping your cells to quickly use up your glycogen and focus on burning fat for energy. In order words, intermittent fasting will help you to get into a metabolic state of ketosis faster than if you depend on only a keto diet.

After achieving ketosis, is the work of intermittent fasting over? Certainly not! You can continue intermittent fasting to ensure a continuous benefit from ketosis as both can help you to:

- Maintain a good level of blood sugar

- Keep your level of cholesterol balanced

- Improve fat loss

- Improve your insulin sensitivity

- Lose weight in a healthy way

Both intermittent fasting and keto are known to sharpen your focus, perk up the memory, and boost mental clarity. Usually, there are often ups and downs in the levels of your blood sugar when you eat high-carbohydrate foods. These ups and downs can cause instability in the energy supply to your brain. However, when you turn to intermittent fasting and keto diet, your body eventually depends on a more consistent source (ketones from fat) for its supply of energy to your brain. This may result in better cognitive functions.

So, is it correct to saythat intermittent fasting always leads to ketosis? No. intermittent fasting doesn't always result in ketosis. Simply fasting for a considerable short window and eating foods that are high in carbohydrate in the eating window may not result in ketosis. And then again, ketosis may not be the goal of everyone who goes into intermittent fasting. However, for those who intend to achieve ketosis, intermittent fasting is a great means to arrive at that destination.

Getting Into Ketosis

Stimulating the metabolic process which breaks down fat into ketone bodies requires that you should be deliberate about what you eat. For the keto diet to work, you need to be committed to the process. Perhaps if you constantly remind yourself that your aim is to tap into the numerous benefits of running your body on fat (instead of glucose), it will make you stick more to your decision to diet using the keto method. You are not doing anything strange when you train (or retrain) your body and brain to focus on broken down fat for energy supply. The purpose of storing fat in your body is so that they will be used. Sticking to the keto diet is using stored fat to your overall health benefit.

For the sake of brevity, I'll quickly highlight some steps for you to take to get your body into ketosis.

1. *Carbohydrate restriction*: a strictly low carbohydrate diet (or keto diet) would usually consist of not more than 20 grams of digestible carbohydrate spread throughout the day. This is one of the most basic steps which may actually be all you need to do to get your body into a metabolic state of ketosis.

2. *Protein restriction*: one common error many

people who want to get into ketosis make is eating too much protein. Excess protein intake would be turned into glucose, and as you do know, glucose is capable of significantly slowing down ketosis. Restrict your intake of protein to a modest amount. I will suggest that you should try to keep your protein intake within the range of 1.5 gram in a day per 1 kilogram of body weight. So if you weigh 80kg (176lb) for example, that would amount to about 120 grams of protein consumption spread throughout your day.

3. *Consume more fat*: you may wonder what difference is there between starvation that results in ketosis and a keto diet that results in ketosis. Here's a major difference. Ketosis as a result of starvation is unsustainable. Ketosis as a result of the keto diet is very sustainable. Starvation causes you to feel very hungry (without the option of eating). On the other hand, the keto diet offers you the chance to eat more fat so that you can feel satiated. Eat healthy fats such as olive oil and butter.

4. *Don't snack*: unless you are hungry, you should avoid snacking. There may be food and snacks at your beck and call, but eating just because there is an abundance of food may hamper weight loss and is likely to inhibit ketosis. Thankfully, there are some healthy keto snacks that are okay to consume provided you are truly hungry.

5. *Combine it with Intermittent Fasting*: intermittent fasting is like the icing on the cake for keto dieting. It is fairly easy to combine, and it enhances the level of ketone. It may also aid in the reversal of type 2 diabetes as well as boost weight loss. However, care should be taken when combining intermittent fasting with keto diet. Do it only if you are sure it is safe for you or is recommended by your doctor.

6. *Workout*: exercising, especially moderate or low impact exercises can have a great impact on your journey to ketosis as it may lead to a moderate increase in the level of ketone.

7. *Get a good sleep*: if you really want your body to get into ketosis, give yourself about 7 hours of good sleep per night. Depriving yourself of sleep (intentionally or unintentionally) may slow down ketosis. Equally, give yourself quality rest.Avoid all forms of stress. Always remember that stress hormones are capable of raising your blood sugar level and that may negatively impact your weight loss and ketosis goal.

Is it Okay to Fast on Keto?

Fasting while you are on the keto diet is usually referred to as "fasting ketosis" or fasting on keto. But is it a good idea to combine intermittent fasting with keto? Is it safe?

Well, if you have no known medical issues, and

if you are certified okay to take on intermittent fasting, then it is also considered safe for you to combine fasting with keto. As earlier mentioned in Chapter 1, intermittent fasting is not focused on what to eat but on when to eat;it is the order of eating, not a diet designed for weight loss. That is one of the major differences between intermittent fasting and keto. However, combining the two may be a major plus as intermittent fasting significantly stimulate the fat burning process of keto.

Also, if you choose to eat your meals in accordance with the ketogenic diet method, you are likely to experience less hunger during fasting because keto diet contains high fat that gives you the feeling of being satiated even with smaller food quantity in your body. Intermittent fasting also opens the way for you to gently introduce keto diet a lot more easily to your body, and it can promote quick results.

Fasting on Keto: The Good

Thereare quite a couple of good effects of combining intermittent fasting with keto dieting. Usually, after the first few weeks of doing the two together, you should be able to get over any unpleasant side effects and begin to see some awesome advantages of the combo.

But wait. There really are side effects of combining the two? Most certainly! Yes, there are. However, they are basically not different from the side effects of intermittent fasting (which is covered in the final chapter of this book). And while it is true that combining fasting and keto have some disadvantages (as if there is anything that doesn't have its own disadvantage), they are ways that you can actually handle these side effects. But for now, let us give our attention to the good and save the bad for later.

Suppression of Appetite and Weight Loss

This seems to be a no-brainer. It is obvious that when you combine intermittent fasting with a keto diet, you are basically reducing your food intake and at the same time promoting the loss of body fat. And your appetite is easily suppressed because your meals consist of foods that are high in fat, and low in carbohydrate. That's a perfect recipe for appetite suppression because the high fat creates a feeling of satiation.

Mental Clarity

Studies have shown that ketones produced in the fat-burning process of keto diet have positive effects on your brain. One of such studies revealed that the ketones released (whether through fasting on keto or simple keto dieting) are capable of crossing over the blood-brain hurdle and supply energy to the brain. They may also provide the benefit of neuroprotection. (US National Library of Medicine, 2008, n.p.).[16]

Improved Energy

The sudden sharp rise in blood sugar can be significantly kept at bay when fasting on keto. This may lead to a stable and steady supply of energy to your body for the entire day. Of course, this benefit takes a while to show up, usually after the first few weeks of fasting on keto.

Preventive Health

Fasting on keto may have health benefits that are more far-reaching and long-term than the issue of weight loss (and I know that it may not be fair to trivialize weight loss as it is very important to many good women – and men too!But considering the long-term preventive health advantages of fasting on keto, weight loss may be a bit way down the line in the grand scheme of things). Some of the preventive health advantages of running your body on fat include a significant reduction in your chances of developing diseases such as Alzheimer's disease,diabetes, and cancer. (US National Library of Medicine, 2013, n.p.).[17]

Fasting on Keto: The Bad

Since intermittent fasting and keto share some similarities, it is quite normal to expect a few similar side effects,especially when combining the two. Keep in mind that these side effects will pass with time (usually within the first few weeks), but if they persist, it is definitely time to seek medical advice.

Keto Flu

Keto flu refers to most of the symptoms I will list in this section. They are generally unpleasant, but they tend to pass after a while. And even though this is supposed to be "the bad" section of fasting on keto, but the effect of keto flu can actually be reduced by introducing fasting into keto diet. In this regard, intermittent fasting on keto diet is actually a plus. This is so because fasting tends to kickoff or stimulates the process of ketosis.

Headaches

Temporary headaches may result from the lowering of insulin as your body cells are acclimating to be dependent on ketones. The likelihood of headaches is also increased by including fasting in your keto regimen.

Fever

Your body is adjusting to a new pattern of eating (and not eating) and at the same time grappling with getting used to high fat and missing its usually high carbohydrate. It is only expected that you may feel a bit feverish during this period of adjustment especially as your body enters ketosis. There are no hard facts or conclusive research on this; however, experiencing fever during fasting on keto may not be unrelated to increased heat as your body burns fat. This may lead to some noticeable increase in your body temperature.

Touchiness

You may not be in the best of moods during your early days of going without food and adjusting to the absence of high carbohydrates and sugar. So you are not a bad woman if you find yourself getting easily irked at your spouse, kids, friends, or neighbors while fasting on keto (just don't let it become a habit!).

Fogginess

Brain fog may result from dips in blood sugar even if you have had enough sleep and rest. So it is not uncommon to experience forgetfulness or a little bit of confusion at the initial stage of fasting on keto.

Now let's take a look at other side effects that may not fall strictly under the keto flu.

Craving and Hunger

Starting an intermittent fasting regimen during keto dieting is very likely to cause some hunger especially if you are new to the whole idea;your body is being pushed to unfamiliar grounds and deprived of its usual calorie intake. Hunger is a natural backlash that occurs in response to this unfamiliar terrain. Your body is already trained or programmed to expect food at certain intervals. One research shows a connection between ghrelin – the appetite hormone – and eating time. Once eating time approaches, ghrelin rings the alarm, and you begin to feel hungry. (Medical Xpress,2009, n.p.).[18]

And because you are low on carbohydrates, your body tends to crave for sweet foods. This craving may be exceptionally high in some people and may lead them to cheat; breaking their fasting untimely and take a quick bite at something sweet.

Cramps

Temporal cramps can result from improper hydration during fasting on keto. Low levels of minerals in your body may also lead to aches in your muscles. Your muscles require proper balance in your electrolytes such as calcium and magnesium – a lack of which may lead to pain or muscle cramps.

Exhaustion

Exhaustion or fatigue is one frequent reason many people can't keep up with fasting on keto before they reach the level of reaping the benefits of ketosis.According to Dr. Anthony Gustin "*Your body needs to produce sugar for energy when fasting, so it begins a process called gluconeogenesis, during which your liver converts non-carbohydrate materials like lactate, amino acids, and fats into glucose. As this occurs, your basal metabolic rate (BMR) uses less energy and your blood pressure and heart rate are lowered. Think of this as your body going into 'power saving mode"'* (Gustin, 2018, n.p.).[19]

This may result in extreme tiredness and weakness. It takes sheer willpower to cross this stage in the fasting on keto journey.

Digestion Issues

Constipation, diarrhea, and frequent bowel movements are symptoms of fasting on keto that may occur during the early days. Stool forms properly when there are enough amounts of food remnants in your stomach (undigested food) which is pushed out as feces. The absence of food in your stomach may lead to smaller or lack of adequate waste material to form proper stool. (Mayo Clinic, 2018, n.p.).[20]Constipation may also result from the absence of fiber in your meals. (US National Library of Medicine, 2010, n.p.).[21]It is also possible to have frequent bowel movements due to some people's sensitivity to some keto foods. Dehydration may also lead to digestive problems.

Bad Breath

Some people call it keto breath, but that label does very little to mask the unpleasant puff that is likely to ooze from your mouth once you begin keto diet. Not to worry; this is not a permanent issue. It happens because of the increased levels of ketone and the release of ketone acetone through the breath. (US National Library of Medicine, 2002, n.p.).[22]

Low Energy

It is very common to feel really drained at the beginning of fasting on keto. As carbohydratesare the major source of energy known by your body before intermittent fasting or keto, it is normal for you to feel a dip in your energy supply at least a few days or weeks when you begin to restrict carbohydrate intake.

Increased or Irregular Heart Rate

There is a possibility of having heart palpitations especially if your blood pressure tends to be on the lower end. Irregular heart rate or increase in heart rate may not be unconnected to a lack of salt and water in your body.

Fasting on Keto: Avoiding the Ugly

Okay, now that we have seen the good and the bad, it's time to avoid the ugly (sounds more like a movie from the mid60s!).

Many of the side effects of fasting on keto will eventually wear off in a couple of weeks if you do take necessary precautions. However, jumping into fasting on keto without proper knowledge is diving headlong for the ugly.Generally, it is recommended that you should keep stress at its barest minimum and get enough rest.During your eating window, make sure to get enough calories into your meals too.

Here are some other recommendations for a less unpleasant sail during your fasting on keto voyage.

Keep Yourself Well-Hydrated

Drink adequate water because you are most likely to flush water from your body making you susceptible to dehydration. It is a great idea to also take mineral-rich broth.

Target Minerals

To regain possibly lost electrolytes, it is recommended that you target foods that are highly nutritious when you break your fast. According to Dr. Anthony Gustin, DC, MS, founder of Perfect Keto,"*Eat plenty of leafy greens, celery, seaweed, cucumber, meat, poultry, fish, avocados and high fat, quality dairy products (if dairy agrees with you). You'll also want to eat plenty of fats such as coconut oil and MCT oil, as they'll keep you satiated without spiking your insulin level.*" (Gustin, 2018, n.p.).[19]

Eat More Salt

Usually, since you are low on carbohydrates, your body flushes out water and in the process, sodium is also lost. It is advisable to slightly increase your salt intake. Not just any salt, but high-quality salt. This is to make sure that the sodium lost from your body during fasting on keto is regained through salt intake.

Use Exogenous Ketones

You may also consider the use of exogenous ketonesto help you switch gently into ketosis at a much quicker rate. Exogenous ketones may help you to speed up the process of ketosis as they supply you with additional ketones as necessary energy for your transition process. When you speed up your ketosis process, there is a good chance of sidestepping some of the side effects of fasting on keto.

Look After Your Overall Well-being

This may seem obvious, but you will be surprised at the number of people who expect that simply deciding to fast on keto is all the health decision they would ever need to make. Give your body some well-deserved care. It has housed you from birth until now, in spite of some not-so-healthy choices you've made in the past. But remember that you are about to combine intermittent fasting with ketosis, so you can't afford to give less attention to your overall health. Fasting on keto may suit you, but if you do not give proper care to your body, you may end up being frustrated. Sleep well, give your body and muscles some movement no matter how light or low-impact, rest well and most importantly eat right when it is time to eat. Do not starve yourself in the guise of fasting on keto. And do not overeat in the guise of breaking your fast.

Take Magnesium Supplements if and only if...

It is a good health practice to keep your electrolytes and hydration at par especially during fasting on keto. One way to maintain a good equilibrium of electrolyte and body water level is by taking magnesium supplements. Nevertheless, if you have any history of kidney problem or you have diarrhea, please consult your doctor or a qualified healthcare provider before attempting to take magnesium supplements.

Weight Loss and Cravings

Dieting for weight loss can be a very difficult plan to follow. And to make matters worse, there is the issue of cravings to deal with too. Advice such as "enjoy in moderation" can be annoying at times, plus it almost always doesn't work. Enjoying your indulgence or cravings in moderation can only work when you have a good grip on them.

So the first course of action is to gain considerable control over your cravings as you journey along to weight loss. When you successfully arrive at your weight loss destination, you can then choose to gradually re-introduce those favorite foods "in moderation." In other words, control comes before moderation, and not the other way round.

A study to support this position observed 367 obese participants for a period of two years while being made to stick to diets that are highly restrictive. Their levels of craving and of course body weight were monitored at the beginning, six months later, and after two years. (US National Library of Medicine, 2017, .n.p.).[23]

The study found that during restriction of calorie intake for the purpose of weight loss, the participants' cravings for a particular type of food were significantly diminished when the eating frequency of those particular foods was reduced. The particular foods were not eaten in lesser quantities; rather, they were eaten less frequently. Simply put, if you are trying to overcome your craving for candy, it will be best to avoid candies completely rather than eating fewer quantities of candy.

This makes perfect sense especially when you are trying to shed off some pounds. You do not get over eating junk foods by taking little bites. You get over them by avoiding them completely. As Lisa DeFazio, R.D., author of *Women's Health Big Book of Soups*, says *"For cravings and junk food, it's like a drug, so the more you eat it, the more you crave it. Even introducing it once a week, gives you that feeling again, releasing dopamine, and leading to that feeling of pleasure."* (DeFazio, 2017, n.p.).[24]

An effective way to completely avoid your cravings is to clean out your cabinet. Don't let them lay around where you can easily access them.

Throw them out and stop buying them.

Another way to greatly reduce the frequency of indulging in your cravings is to get rid of the trigger that is linked to your craving. For example, watching TV may trigger in you a need to crunch on some of your favorite candy. In that case, avoid watching TV in order to not trigger the automatic need to reach out and grab some candy. But then, that may be a difficult option. However, you can choose to substitute the candy (or whatever your cravings are) with a healthy alternative. Just remember to keep it very minimal so that you don't create a craving for another thing altogether.

The Psychology Behind Food Cravings

Perhaps an understanding of the psychology behind why you crave all the "wrong" foodswill help you with your weight loss goals. Your intention to lose weight may be noble, but your cravings don't know that, and they are hell-bent on keeping you from reaching your goal. But understanding why this is so will give you a good head start.

Sensory Cues

Images of food, advertisements, and the delicious aroma of food can trigger in us the need to eat whatever is causing such trigger irrespective of what junks or calories they contain.

Gherlinstirs up your brain to notice more of food cues when you are hungry. Our brain tends to seek out unhealthy foods when we are hungry. (US National Library of Medicine, 2017, n.p.).[25]In some studies, participants were shown images of foods that are high in calories. They reported that the food cues aroused in them the desire to eat. This showed up in participants' craving and salivation. (British Journal of Nutrition, 2008, n.p.).[26]

What this simply means is that foods that are high in calorie are likely to draw more attention and pose a serious challenge to people who wish to lose weight, especially if they go without food for significant amount of time to make them hungry.

The "Off-limits" Label Appears More Enticing

"Do not eat this or that," has an ironic way of making you want to "eat this or that." But why is this so? This may not be unconnected to an innate desire to try out things that are "off-limits." It appears our minds place a big bull's eye or a conspicuous mark on the foods that we are supposed to avoid. These "off-limits" foods become even more desirous and we are more drawn to them simply by depriving us of them. (Science Direct, 2011, n.p.).[27]

Perhaps it is the idea of "giving up" associated with dieting that makes gratifying foods more difficult to let go. One study which has participants that eat chocolates on a rather frequent basis asked them to give up eating chocolate for one whole week. The research shows that images of chocolate or foods that are high in calorie became more appealing or noticeable to these participants. The restriction on chocolate has made them more inclined to desire foods that are high in calorie than the participants who were not deprived of eating chocolates. (Plos One, 2014, n.p.).[28]

Furthermore, a study shows that participants who were asked to eat "off-limits" food after being deprived of it for a while, consumed higher amounts of calories. (US National Library of Medicine, 2008, n.p.).[29]

What this comes down to is this: staying away from desirable or pleasurable foods creates a high attraction for that food due to your brain's (and body's) reaction to the idea of being deprived of your pleasure.

There's No Point in Continuing. I've Broken the Rules Already

With all the rigid rules about what to eat, how to eat it, when to eat it, and in what quantity to eat it, many people find it difficult to follow with through diet plans (no matter how good the plans are). The thing with all these rules is that violating them (even in a little way) is capable of leading the dieter completely off course. Studies have shown that when people believe that they have broken the strict rules of their diet plan, they tend to continue down that path or at least repeat the violation. Their thinking goes along the lines of "I've broken the rules already, so there's no point sticking to the rules." This is what researchers refer to as the "what-the-hell effect." (Selig, M. 2011, n.p.).[30]

In reality, a few missteps in dieting may not cause any significant negative impact, but the negative psychological impact on the dieter may be the cause of derailment from the diet plan. This negative psychological impact can set off a feeling of guilt or stress. In the long run, the dieter may find his or herself overeating – an effect associated with guilt or stress. (Psychology & Health, 2015, p. 203-217).[31]

Having considered the psychology behind cravings, you should not beat yourself up for "breaking the rules." You are human, and rules are meant to be... well, let's just say, humans are not too good at keeping to rules a hundred percent of the time. So if you break a rule, it's not time to throw your hands in the air and give up: "I'm never going to shed off this damn weight!" Simply dust yourself up, and try again. The psychological effect of failing at dieting (or giving in to craving) may lead you to gain back whatever weight you have began to lose.

Your Age and Cravings

Generally, women have unusually strong cravings when they become pregnant. This is due to abnormal levels of hormonal rush. These types of cravings are only temporal and will subside after childbirth.

Thankfully, cravings seem to decrease as we grow older. Perhaps it is because our palates have been caused to experience a wide range of different foods, or it is due to some psychological reasons. In order to discover the connection between age and cravings, researchers conducted a study of 105 persons between the ages of 6 to 23. (Freedhoff, 2013, n.p.).[32]

The participants were exposed to pictures of sweet and unhealthy foods as they were being scanned (fMRI). The study found that children have the greatest yearning for unhealthy and sweet foods than the rest of the participants.

So as you grow older, you may be able to handle your cravings better, however; your metabolism may also slow down with age.

Tips on How to Not Give In to Cravings

Fighting off cravings may be challenging but it can be done. Below, I have outlined a few tips that you may find useful to effectively combat food cravings. Let me quickly point out that these tips are not quick fixes. Consistency in using these tips is what pays off in the long run. So do not expect your cravings to vanish overnight because of a "magical" tip you applied. It doesn't work that way. You are dealing with a deeply ingrained (almost biological) pattern of behavior; therefore, it will take time to course-correct.

Drink Enough Water

"Drink enough water" seems to be the classic advice for handling food cravings and it is for a good reason (after all, your body is largely made up of water). Sometimes when you think you are hungry, you may actually just be thirsty. So, the next time you feel like eating in between meals or snacking, reach for a glass of water instead and gulp down a large amount of water. You may be pleasantly surprised that the craving has passed because thirst may be the actual issue, not hunger.

Drinking enough water may also be a good way to significantly cut down appetite. With low appetite comes low cravings and may ultimately lead to weight loss.

Stress Less

One factor that may also increase your cravings is stress. When you are stressed, there is more likelihood for you to consume foods that have considerably large amounts of calories which can lead to cravings. This is especially true in many women. Additionally, stress can also raise the level of cortisol hormone in your blood. Cortisol is capable of causing weight gain particularly around the region of the belly.

Keep your stress level as low as possible especially if you are interested in sticking to your weight loss goal and avoiding food cravings. Both mental and physical stress should be avoided as much as possible.

Plan Your Meals

Planning what to eat for the entire day or even a whole week can be a great way to reduce cravings. Planning your meals has a way of letting your mind close the chapter on thinking about food. It's like saying "let's get this done and over with." When you already take the time to draw out exactly what to eat at what time and in what quantity, it takes your mind away from thinking about food for the rest of the day (or week). It also removes the element of uncertainty and impulsiveness that may push you into taking a quick bite of your favorite snack every now and then.

So, take the time to browse for some awesome tips on how to plan your meals (that's if you don't already know how to do it), or speak to a dietician to help you work out a sustainable (doable) plan for your meal that will suit your particular goal.

Remember, one of the reasons planning meals don't seem to work or following through with planned meals seems to be cumbersome is because people become impractical when planning meals. The goal is to make it sustainable over a long time so that you can see improvement in your eating habit which will ultimately lead to improved health. Being too rigid or unreasonable can cause burnouts. For example, completely removing carbohydrates from your meals at a go may not be a sustainable and doable thing. It may work for a few days, but keeping it up may not be feasible. You have to approach this the way someone with a "bad" habit or an addiction would – a gradual process of elimination (eating your favorite food less frequently) so that your body can get used to the absence of the foods that you crave.

Increase Your Protein Intake

Adding more protein to your meals may help to curb the need to overeat. Foods that are rich in protein can reduce your appetite, effectively leading to less desire for snacking. If you want to reduce nighttime snacking, you may want to consider eating more protein-rich foods.

Sleep More

Inadequate sleep may be linked to disruptions in the hormone that signals hunger. When you deprive yourself of enough sleep, it is likely to cause improper regulation of hunger which may,in turn, lead to more cravings.

Give yourself enough time in bed and possibly get extra sleep to keep your cravings at bay.

Chapter 8: Autophagy

What it is and What it Does

~~∞~~

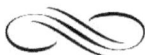

Your body eats itself! Yes, I know. It sounds weird but it's true. Autophagy is a process (a good process, by the way) which your body uses to remove broken cells and toxic materials to make way for better cells. It is a way the body adapts to rejuvenate itself.

When loosely translated, the "auto" in autophagy means self and "phagy" means to eat. So autophagy enables your body to eat cells that it considers no more useful to its well-being.

With time, there is a buildup of spoilt proteins, dead cell parts, and harmful particles that hamper the smooth functioning of your body. This buildup increases the rate at which your body ages, amplifies your chances of developing cancer, stimulates dementia, and increases the chances of getting other diseases that come with aging. To protect itself from the harmful effects of this buildup, the body cleanses itself through the process of autophagy.

Naomi Whittel aptly describes autophagy with

this analogy. *"Think of your body as a kitchen. After making a meal, you clean up the counter, throw away the leftovers, and recycle some of the food. The next day, you have a clean kitchen. This is autophagy doing its thing in your body, and doing it well."* (Bullet Proof, 2018, n.p.).[33]

But what happens as you grow older is that the cleaning process of autophagy slows down and bits and pieces of "cell crumbs," scattered "protein parts," and a whole other mess are left unattended due to inefficiency that comes with age.

Nevertheless, you can stimulate and keep autophagy well activated and ready to clean up as effectively and efficiently as it used to. Stress-inducing activity (such as prolong hunger or famine) can activate autophagy and keep it on top gear. This will decrease the rate at which you age, decrease inflammation, and improve your body's overall well-being.

Autophagy: The Science Behind It

A study conducted by Newcastle University found that because humans learned to adapt and respond in better ways to biological stressors, we gradually advanced over time to live longer. (Newcastle University, 2018, n.p.).[34]This ability to react well to stressors is as a result of *"adaptations in a protein known as p62 that induces autophagy."* (Bullet Proof, 2018, n.p.).[35]

Let's take a quick peek into what goes on inside our cells when autophagy is activated. As soon as p62 notices metabolic wastes that are capable of causing damages to the cell, it stimulates autophagy which begins the cleaning process. Our good protein friend, the p62, clears away any damaged cell or residual parts of wastes that are lying around in your body constituting nuisances. This clearing puts your body in a good position to effectively tackle any biological stress. The work of p62 on your cells is what keeps your cells (and byextension, you) strong, healthy, and youthful.

The study I earlier referred to, conducted by Newcastle University, observed that some organisms such as fruit flies do not have the ability that humans have to handle biological stress. In order to confirm this, the researchers genetically altered some fruit flies and gave them the human version of our good protein friend, the p62. What they found was pretty amazing. The genetically altered fruit flies were able to live longer even under uncomfortable conditions (stress). Dr. VicktorKorolchuk, the lead author of the study, gave this succinct conclusion, *"This tells us that abilities, like sensing stress and activating protective processes like autophagy, may have evolved to allow better stress resistance and a longer lifespan"* (Bullet Proof, 2018, n.p.).[35]

Autophagy: The Benefits

Leaving worn out and damaged cells in the body can lead to Alzheimer's Disease and possibly cancer. When there is a buildup of damaged protein cells in the brain, it is likely to result in Alzheimer's Disease. This being true, it is only logical to see how it is possible for autophagy to remove unwanted or damaged protein cells and in turn reduce the chances of developing Alzheimer's Disease.

Autophagy is known to have the following benefits:

- *Reduction in the rate of aging*: accumulation of damaged cells and wastes causes an acceleration in the rate at which we age. When you activate autophagy, it slows down the process, and you age gracefully.

- *Keeps neurodegenerative diseases in check*: neurodegenerative diseases such as Alzheimer's Disease, are kept at bay when the cleaning process of autophagy is fully functional.

- *Increased functionality*: autophagy promotes your overall health and enhances your general body functions.

- *Perk up your muscle performance*: during exercises, there is a risk of injury to your muscles, and this needs to be repaired. Autophagy will help in improving the damaged components in your muscles.

Other benefits includea reduction in inflammation and improved skin complexion.

Intermittent Fasting and Autophagy

There are two ways fasting helps our body. First, fasting stimulates autophagy which essentially rids the body of harmful and unused parts.Secondly, it boosts growth hormones which signal our body to manufacture fresh parts to keep us running smoothly.

Basically, fasting deprives the body of nutrients long enough to activate autophagy.But does autophagy works in women the same way it does in men? Does the sex of the individual matter?

Well, intermittent fasting is known to stimulate neuronal autophagy. However, while this may be true for men, it may not be completely true for some women. A study shows that neurons in males may respond to food deprivation (or fasting) by activating autophagy. Nevertheless, the female neurons respond to starvation or fasting by opposing autophagy. *"The role of autophagy during starvation is both sex- and tissue-dependent. Thus, during starvation, neurons from males more readily undergo autophagy and die, whereas neurons from females mobilize fatty acids, accumulate triglycerides, form lipid droplets, and survive longer."* (US National

Library of Medicine, 2009, n.p.).[36]

This, however, does not mean autophagy is not good for women. It simply means that males are likely to achieve a faster result with autophagy than females. Moreover, having a little resistance to autophagy is not such an awful thing. According to the *Journal of Cardiovascular Translational Research,* some diseases have been found to sneak up on the human body using the cover of autophagy to remove both healthy and unhealthy cells. And the good news is, women are less likely to contract these diseases. (Journal of Cardiovascular Translational Research, 2014, p.182-191).[37]

Chapter 9: Fasting Plus Exercise – Good Combo?

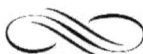

O kay, so you've made up your mind to start fasting and you are really fired up and ready to go. But what about workouts? Can you still exercise during fasting? If yes, what types of exercises are recommended? And won't you lose muscle if you exercise during fasting? Is it really safe? What does science say about combining fasting and exercising?

Well, you may want to slow down a bit with the

questions, let's take them one after the other.

Is It Okay To Exercise During Intermittent Fasting?

The short answer is: yes, it is safe to exercise during fasting, but it is not safe for everyone.

Now, let take a look at the long answer.

It depends on the individual, the type of intermittent fasting (or fasting in general), and the type of exercise. Add to the list, the mental, physical, and psychological states of the individual and you will have a fairly good idea of why it is difficult to box everyone into one category with a clear-cut answer.

There are studies and counter-studies on the subject of exercising while fasting. The reason for such disagreements may not be unrelated to the uniqueness of each individual. Even though we may all look alike and have the same basic physiology, there are several unique indices that may be different for each individual. And a woman's body is especially more complex. The varying studies nonetheless, there are some facts that you need to understand before combining intermittent fasting and exercising.

Let us consider these facts in a nutshell. While it is true that you may burn a significantly higher amount of fat during exercises combined with intermittent fasting, it is also possible to reduce the rate of your metabolism if the fasting is for a very long period (for example, if you continue to combine fasting and exercises for up to a month or more).

There is also the possibility of not being at your "A-game" when you exercise while fasting. This is true for many people. It is also possible that you will not build up your muscles (even if you don't lose them). However, you may at least be able to maintain your muscles.

Recommended Exercises During Fasting

Below are some low-impact exercises that I would recommend for women who want to combine exercise with intermittent fasting. Although they are considered low-impact, it doesn't make them ineffective. On the contrary, your joints are probably going to love you more for using them especially during fasting because they are gentler on your body. They are safer and easier without giving you concern about injuries and too much strain, yet there can be used as a good way to give your heart some real pumping.

1. *Yoga*: this practice has various poses that are great at making you experience the burnout without feeling the pain. So check out some nice poses that appeal to you and include them in your workout routines.

2. *Cycling*: this is another good way of giving your joints some workout devoid of pains. Get a hold of some good old bicycle and ride for about 30 minutes to give your joints some great exercise.

3. *Strength Training*: there are several strength training workouts that are considered low-impact. But low-impact or not, they are a great way to break a sweat.

4. *Rowing*:30 minutes of rowing is sure to give your core, arms, legs, and back some great workout. Remember not to overdo this as your aim is low-impact workouts.

5. *Tai Chi*: if you are looking for an easy way to improve your flexibility consider Tai Chi. It's flowing, easy, and gentle movements ensure that your exercises are not strenuous and it may even have an added benefit of dispelling headaches.

6. *Roller-skating*: take off some stress from your limbs as you glide easily along pavements while burning some calories. Be sure to wear protective gear to prevent injuries during a fall. It is probably best to skip skating if you don't know or if you have forgotten how to apply the brakes!

7. *Walking*: give your body some movement by taking a walk. You may choose to add ankle weight or walk up a hilly or steep terrain to get your heart pumping faster.

8. *Hiking*:if walking is too leisurely for you, get your

boots and do some hiking! Remember, you are combining this with fasting, so keep things simple by hiking on easy terrains.

9. *Kayaking*: give your arms some workout to improve your arm muscles and flexibility. It can also improve your core even without crunches or sit-ups.

10. *Golfing*: while some people may put off golfing as a sport for only professional golfers or for retired people, it is actually a good sport for everyone who wants to use swinging to get in some great body movement. You can also choose to skip the use of a golf cart and instead, walk across the golf course; effectively combining two low-impact exercises – golfing and walking.

11. *Rock Climbing*: this has a way of giving your muscles some serious workout as it involves measured and meticulous movements. Although your muscles are being seriously worked on, you will hardly feel any suddenexertion. Remember to take necessary safety precautions before attempting rock climbing.

12. *Snowshoeing*: for a good body-friendly exercise, try strapping on your snowshoes and walk on snow. This is more of an exercise than a leisurely walk along the pavement.

13. *Swimming*: with a combined benefit of improving the functioning of your lungs and

giving more strength to your shoulders, this low-impact exercise is really fun and also keeps your body cool and hydrated when done during your fasting window.

14. *Step Aerobics*: when done for about an hour, it has the combined effects of a good mid-distance run and a great cardio workout. And it has the bonus of excluding all the strenuous poundings.

15. *Pilates*: if you are looking to achieve a tough core give this a shot. It is a great way to take your flexibility to a whole new level with the added benefit of being easy on your joints.

16. *Stair-Master*: going up and down a flight of stairs can be a good way to knock the wind out of you whenever you feel heavy. But be sure to keep it moderate considering that you are on a fast.

17. *Total-body Resistance Exercises*: this is a type of workout that uses a strap suspension system to perform a total-body resistance exercise. Your joint may not feel the brunt of this exercise, but the rest of your body is sure to feel the pressure.

18. *Dancing*: dancing is gentle on the body, plus it could be sexy especially when dancing with a partner. It's like combining work and pleasure. Just don't get into acrobats and break dance.

19. *Skiing*: propelling yourself with poles across a plain snowfield is a great way to keep your muscles working, heart pumping, and your body

warm even in the freezing weather. This is an awesome way to give yourself some light-pressured exercise.

The Exception

Except based on a medical recommendation, I do not encourage rigorous or strenuous exercises during fasting. If you are a woman who does heavy lifting, I suggest you eat your meal after 30 minutes of heavy lifting or thereabout. That is to say, if you must lift heavy weights while fasting, ensure to time your exercises towards the end of your fasting window. And when you do eat, focus on foods that contain quick-assimilating proteins. According to Dr. Niket Sonpal, an Adjunct Assistant Professor of Clinical Medicine at Touro College of Osteopathic Medicine, *"And if you do heavy lifting, it's important for your body to have protein after the workout to aid with regeneration"* (Sonpal, 2018, n.p.).[38]

If you must engage in strenuous exercises, I would recommend that you allow your body to get used to low-impact exercises before you gradually up the stake. So, yes, you can do high-impact workouts during fasting on the condition that you have given your body a considerable amount of time to adjust to intermittent fasting with low-impact exercises.

Always remember that it is important to maintain a good blood sugar level. Doing anything to negatively impact your blood sugar level may result in feeling lightheaded or dizzy. If you feel dizzy during your exercise routines while you are on intermittent fasting, please stop the routine immediately and seek medical attention as soon as possible.

Fasting Plus Exercise: Burn Muscles or Build Muscles?

First off, let's get something clear. There is a difference between building or adding muscle and maintaining muscle mass. Some people usually use the two interchangeably, but they are not the same. While the former means increasing your lean muscles, the latter is keeping the existing muscles intact – not burning them, and not building them. Furthermore, there's a huge misconception about losing weight and losing muscles. The fact that you are beginning to observe a decrease in your overall body weight does not automatically translate into burning of fat.

If weight gain or loss is your goal, then you need to focus on the type of food you eat and when you eat them (dieting or intermittent fasting). If reducing or increasing your muscle mass is your goal, then you need to focus on the exercises you do. And you have the option of combining it with any type of fasting that suits your goal. As Dr. Jason Fung, puts it, *"you can't out-run a bad diet. You can't eat your way to more muscle"* (Fung,

2017, n.p.).[39]

So if you are concerned about building your muscles or you are worried that fasting will make you lose your muscles, there is a simple way to handle that. Do more exercises. Do not stress yourself about what fasting or your meals are going to do to your muscles. Give your attention wholly to exercising. And if you can combine exercisewith fasting, you may likely get more than one benefit.

Now to the main question: do we burn muscles when fasting and exercising at the same time?

The answer to this is very simple. No. You do not burn muscles when exercising whether you are fasting or not. You may burn fat which may lead to weight loss, and that is expected. But while you may not increase your muscle mass during exercises, you do not burn muscle.

This may sound new to you, but it is common sense. Your body stores up surplus energy as body fat so that it can use them when the need arises. When you do not give your body energy supply from your meals, it should naturally turn to its "reserve tank" and feed itself or energize itself using the stored fat. It doesn't make any sense for your body to resort to burning your muscles for energy when it has a tank full of energy reserve. As Dr. Jason puts it, *"Protein is functional tissue and has many purposes other than energy storage, whereas fat is specialized for energy storage.*

Would it not make sense that you would use fat for energy instead of protein?... That is kind of like storing firewood for heat. But as soon as you need heat, you chop up your sofa and throw it into the fire. That is completely idiotic and that is not the way our bodies are designed to work." (Fung, 2017, n.p.).[39]

Maintaining Muscle Mass

A study which showed interesting findings about this question was published by the US National Library of Medicine, and titled: *The protein-retaining effects of growth hormone during fasting involve inhibition of muscle-protein breakdown* (US National Library of Medicine, 2011, n.p.). [40]

The study revealed that retaining muscle mass is possibly linked to our growth hormones. As we already know for a long time (and as acknowledged by the study), during fasting periods, there is usually a considerable reduction in the breakdown of muscles. With the aid of a drug, the growth hormones of the subjects of the research were stifled during fasting, and their muscles were closely monitored to observe any breakdown in the muscles. Interestingly, there was a significant increase (about 50%) in the breakdown of muscles simply by repressing the growth hormone. This strongly suggests that during fasting, growth hormones have a vital part in retaining lean muscle.Our bodies are intelligent enough to preserve its muscles during fasting. When we eat, that is, when we are not fasting, the growth hormone supports our body to rebuild whatever muscles was broken down during fasting. It is a common mistake to view muscle loss from the angle of breakdown without giving due consideration to the fact that the body rebuilds it when we eat food.

All this goes to show that our muscles are not used up when we fast. Fat stored in our bodies are used up to keep us functioning well. The body does not use protein as glucose;it uses fat as energy when you stop giving it food from your meals (fasting).

When we fast, there are several changes in our hormones that signals our adrenalin to shoot up to provide more vigor, and our fatty acids burn more to provide more power, plus our growth hormones ensure the maintenance of lean muscles.

Benefits of Exercising During Fasting

For those who are already into exercising regularly, it may be an added benefit to combine it with fasting. This is likely to increase the benefits of your workouts with the added benefit of fasting.

While a lot of women tend to combine fasting with exercise for the main goal of losing weight (some are actually obsessed about sexy curves), and a lot of men tend to do same with the main goal of building muscles (the Schwarzenegger look), there are even far more benefits of combining exercises with fasting than mere weight loss and muscle building.

Exercising during fasting is a way to make you burn more body fat. This is so because the sympathetic nervous system in your body which is in charge of burning of fat is activated by the absence of food and exercising. This combo increases the impact of some catalysts in your body to breakdown glycogen and body fat.

There have been studies that show the positive effect of exercising during fasting. One of such scientific findings show that there are significant drops in the level body fat and body weight when fasting is combined with exercising. (Mercola, 2013, n.p.).[41]

Furthermore, combining fasting with exercising is likely to result in acute oxidative stress. This is very good for your muscles as they are necessary for maintaining and improving your muscles' resilience to the stress caused by too much oxygen in your cells. Your muscles are likely to age much more slowly when you exercise while fasting. This combo may also activate a special process in your body that revivifies and reuses the tissues of your muscles and the cells of your brain. In other words, this is like keeping the tissues of your muscles, as well as the cells of your brain youthful, biologically speaking. (Mercola, 2011, n.p.).[42]

Some other benefits of exercising during intermittent fasting are:

- Increase growth hormone

- Inhibit depression

- Perk up your body constituents

Tips to Staying Safe While Exercising During Fasting

While it may be considered safe to exercise during fasting, it is important to remember a few tips that would ensure that you remain in the "safe zone." Below are some of the tips to keep in mind.

Pick the Right Time

Give careful thoughts to when you want to time your exercises while you are fasting. Should you exercise during the fasting window, or after the fasting window (that is, during the eating window)?

If you work out very well on an empty stomach, it may be best if you exercise during the fasting window. And if you are great with exercises shortly after eating, then you may probably opt for exercising after the fasting window. And yes, eating shortly before exercising does not necessarily impact your workout in any way.

If you prefer eating before exercising, that is, having meals during the eating window before exercising, it is necessary to shift the time for your exercises to fall into the eating window. This will help your body to maintain a good nutritional level.

Please note that the suggestion about timing your exercises to fall during or after the fasting window is a broad generalization. Do remember that there is no one size fits all.

Keep Yourself Hydrated

Fasting – the type recommended in this book – does not stop you from drinking water. Water is very important if you intend to fast and exercise at the same time. So keep yourself very hydrated at all times.

Don't Push Yourself

You may have to step back a bit from your usual workout goals.Too much strain may not work well for you during this period. In any case, if you begin to feel a bit dizzy when exercising, it is a good time to take a short break.

Watch Your Electrolyte Level

Since you can take liquid during intermittent fasting, it is recommended to focus on keeping your electrolyte level up. Drink liquids that are rich in electrolytes such as coconut water. Sports drinks may not be the perfect choice for you during fasting if you intend to exercise, because they contain high sugar.

Macronutrients are Important Too

What macronutrients are you consuming in the periods long before your exercises? It is important to ensure you get a good amount of macronutrients into your meal the day preceding your exercise. This also applies to the eating window immediately after the fasting.

The Type of Fast Matters

The type of intermittent fasting you undertake will determine the type of exercise you should engage in. Longer fasts such as the 24 hour fast or One Meal A Day (OMAD) that has a very small eating window may not be the best fit for intense exercises. If you are going to be fasting for longer periods, you may want to consider performing simple exercises such as restorative yoga or walking.

Finally...Read The Signs

Your body gives you constant signals about what's going on within you. Pay close attention to it. It may be okay to combine fasting and exercise for other people, but it may not be okay for you. Ultimately, it is all up to you and for goodness sake, use some common sense too. In any case, I strongly suggest that you listen to your body and talk with your healthcare expert or doctor so that you can take an informed decision.

Chapter 10: Intermittent Fasting: Side Effects and How to Troubleshoot

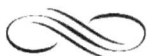

∞

There's hardly any known human practice that does not have some form of side effect. Intermittent fasting is not an exception to that rule either. I am aware that a lot of diehard fans of intermittent fasting may not want to admit there are side effects, but this book will be imbalanced if we focus only on the benefits without presenting some of the side effects.

These side effects are real; they are not imaginary. It is possible to fast without experiencing some of these side effects, but then again, that may be due to individual differences. You may experience some, all, or none of the side effects mentioned in this book. Whatever your particular experience, it is important to note these effects and learn how to troubleshoot them. Let me also add that many of the side effects of intermittent fasting are usually felt at the beginning of the process. As your body gets used to the process, it is likely that the side effects may subside. Give your body time to adjust and learn how to troubleshoot some of these side effects to help you handle them while your body acclimates to your new eating pattern.

Without downplaying the many benefits of intermittent fasting, here are some of the side effects you may encounter during your journey with intermittent fasting.

Headaches

It is not uncommon to have headaches every once in a while as you begin your fasting regimen. It is probably linked to a decrease in the level of your blood sugar. Headaches may also be linked to the activity of your brain in releasing of stress hormones – a common occurrence during fasting. Dehydration may also be a cause of a headache during intermittent fasting.

To Troubleshoot: Always make certain that you stay well hydrated by drinking adequate amounts of water. Remember not to overdo this – drinking too much water may lead to imbalance in your body water and mineral ratio. Also, keep away from stress as much as possible.

Hunger

After several years of conditioning your body to eat three, four, or even five times a day, it is only normal for you to feel very hungry if you alter that eating frequency and pattern. Your body is already programmed to expect food at the usual times you have your meals and take your snacks. The hormone in charge of making you feel hungry – ghrelin – is always on high alert during your scheduled eating time to make you feel hungry so that you placate it with some food. So, when you begin fasting, definitely ghrelin will continue to ring its alarm bell especially at the usual times you eat your meals, and you may feel really, really hungry.At such times (especially as you are just starting out with fasting), it takes real mental strength to tough it out. The first few days will really take its toll on you, but if you stick to your commitment (within reason),you will soon get to the point where rushing to grab a bite immediately after your fasting window ends will be a thing of the past.

To Troubleshoot:Water may keep hunger at bay. Whenever you feel hungry, drink water or liquids that do not contain calories;they can help in suppressing hunger. Additionally, make sure you keep yourself busy at home or at work. Do some simple, low-impact exercises (especially at the beginning of your fasting), and also make sure you catch some quality sleep. It may also help if you eat enough healthy fats, carbohydrates, and proteins the day before your fasting. By "eat enough" I do not mean large quantity. I am simply suggesting the quality of food to eat.

Cravings

The thing about cravings is that it is partly psychological and partly biological. Because of your previous conditioning to eat at certain intervals, deciding all of a sudden to change that pattern will naturally make you crave food at the usual interval. It is psychologically normal. Here's an example to drive home the point. Let us suppose you love apples, but you are asked to never eat apples again, you will most likely feel more inclined to eat apples! Being used to food, your body will make you feel like eating even more than before because it is aware that you are being "deprived" of food. You may also notice that you yearn for carbohydrates or sugar. That's because your body is intensifying its search for glucose.

To Troubleshoot:Distract yourself from thinking about eating;keep your mind busy. When you get to your eating window, it is okay to pamper yourself a bit with a little of those things your body is craving for so as to douse the longing.

Low Energy

It is not completely out of place to feel a bit lethargic during fasting. After all, your body has been conditioned for a long time to get its supply of fuel from your regular meals, so for the first few weeks, it is very likely that you will feel less energized.

To Troubleshoot: Do all you possibly can to keep your activities as low-keyed as possible. Do not push yourself or test your limits especially in the early days. Spending extra time in bed relaxing or sleeping may also keep your energy level up.

Bloating, Constipation, and Heartburn

Although not a common side effect, heartburn may occur as a result of stomach acids produced in order to aid digestion. When there is no food to be digested in the stomach, it may cause heartburn.

Bloating which derives from constipation may also be side effects of intermittent fasting. This too,can really cause some major discomfort.

To Troubleshoot: Drinking good amounts of water should take care of bloating and constipation. For heartburns, it usually passes with time. So do not fret, just drink enough water and avoid eating too manyspicy foods when you eat. Also, try propping up yourself when going to sleep. However, if any of these side effects persist, it is best to consult your healthcare provider.

Bad Temper

You have food, but you don't want to eat, so you are hungry and your cravings are tempting you to break your fast. Add to that the feeling of sluggishness, exhaustion, and the fact that your blood sugar level has taken a nosedive, and it all equals to bad temper!It is okay to feel easily irritable during intermittent fasting because it seems everything in your body system is going out of whack.

To Troubleshoot: Stay away from people and

situations that you consider annoying. They'll just aggravate your edginess. Give your attention to things – situations and people – that easily bring happiness to you. You have to be deliberate about this. Look for happy things and give them your undivided attention. Gratitude and appreciation may also help to keep your mind on happy thoughts.

Feeling Cold

Fasting may cause your blood sugar level to drop and this can lead to making you feel cold. Also, during fasting, there is an increase in the flow of blood to your internal fat storage. This increase in the flow of blood causes your fat to be moved to where it can be used up as energy. This whole process may leave areas of your body with less fat storage (for example, your toes and fingers) feeling cold.

To Troubleshoot: Take a hot shower, drink something hot (perhaps tea or coffee), stay in warm places, and put on some warm clothing, etc.

Frequent Urination

It is only expected that you visit the bathroom frequently since you are drinking larger amounts of water. You need it – your body needs the water, so you can't avoid drinking it except you want to dehydrate yourself which is very dangerous for your health.

To Troubleshoot: Wherever you are, always stay close to a restroom, a toilet, or a bathroom!There really is no shortcut for this one. You should use a bathroom when the need arises, period.

Binging

For beginners, there is a high chance of eating too much when they break their fast. For some, it may be due to being really hungry that they become too eager to shovel food into their stomach and end up binging. And for others, it may be that they have heard that intermittent fasting helps you restrict your calorie intake during the fasting window, so they can eat as manycalories as they want during the eating window. This type of thinking may end up causing frustration especially if you are looking to lose some weight as a side bonus of intermittent fasting. Calories do matter even in intermittent fasting. You will simply undo during the eating window, what you have done during the fasting window if you overeat especially if weight loss is of concern to you.

To Troubleshoot: Plan your meals ahead of the eating window and make sure you stick to the plan. Your plan should include the type of meal as well as the portion or size to be eaten.

It's Not a Diehard Affair

Do have it at the back of your mind that intermittent fasting is not a do-or-die affair. There is a place for quitting even in the middle of your fasting window. There is no rule of thumb that says, "Once you begin fasting, don't break it until the fasting window is over, even when you are dying!" It is important to pay attention to your body to know when these side effects are yelling at the top of their lungs for you to quit. Listen and quit (at least for that day). But do make sure that you are really quitting because of a side effect, and not because you simply want to cheat or you are too lazy to follow through with your commitment.

Conclusion

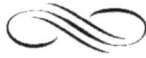

There's a lot of misgivings about fasting; but that's all there are – misgivings. A proper understanding about fasting will eliminate all doubts and fear about fasting. This book has attempted to address most of the doubts and fears associated with this pattern of eating that many are yet to come to terms with.

Although weight loss may be a resultant effect of intermittent fasting, I encourage you to approach intermittent fasting from a different perspective. Look at the various health benefits linked to intermittent fasting and make an informed decision (with the help of your healthcare provider).

If weight loss or weight gain is your main motivation, I suggest you look at your diet – what types of food do you eat? What's your calorie intake? You can combine this with intermittent fasting as a means to restrict calorie intake, but not as a means to get intermittent fasting to reduce your weight (by itself).

If your goal is to build muscles, I would suggest you look at workout routines that are designed to impact your muscles. You can choose to combine these workout routines with intermittent fasting if you wish to exercise on an empty stomach. This has its benefits too but do understand that intermittent fasting alone cannot develop your muscles.

Maintaining a healthy eating habit is important because no matter the amount of fat your body burns during fasting, if you go back to eat junks after your fasting window, your work done is probably equal to zero. Binging after fasting does no good either. This perhaps is the proper role of water and fluid intake as an essential part of your fasting routine. Drinking enough water or fluids during the fasting window and combining that with a good meal design(nutrient-rich foods as well as portions) will probably solve the problem of binging. Eat healthy (intermittent fasting or not) to remain healthy.

This book was written to help people (women especially) who want to heal their bodies with intermittent fasting (weight loss is a bonus). Women who have issues with insulin resistance and diabetes are encouraged to take a look at intermittent fasting in the hope that it may provide an alternative way of helping them deal with these issues. Activating autophagy in order to reverse aging or help you age gracefully is another benefit of intermittent fasting and a major focus of this book.

I encourage you to enjoy life and all the fun it has to offer. Intermittent fasting is not an excuse to live like a prisoner in your own body. Put obsessions about weight loss behind you. Stop giving too much thought to having the perfect shape, or perfect health. As you engage in fasting, your progress may be a bit slow in coming; don't fret. Remember, there may be some level of truth to the idea of mind over matter. And this may be the reason why many people who fret too much about their weight end up gaining more weight. The psychological stress you put yourself through by worrying is capable of triggering your stressors which may inhibit any further progress towards your intermittent fasting goals. Cut yourself some slack. Do not engage yourself in self-pity or beating up on yourself if you misstep or falter once in a while. You are not a robot. You are human, and humans do make mistakes. Even though it is a great idea to be committed to your fasting routine, remember that the routines are created for you, and not you for the routines. Bottom line: let the process be an enjoyable one for you, if not, you probably may not also enjoy the results.

I know I may have sounded like a broken record to some people, but I still must repeat that you should have a talk with your doctor before applying any of the suggestions or recommendations provided in this book. This is not a one size fits all book. Intermittent fasting is not something to be scared of; it is both safe and normal, but it is not for everyone.

Works Cited

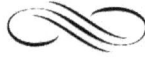

1. Spector, D. (2018). *Here's how many days a person can survive without water.* Retrieved from https://www.businessinsider.com/how-many-days-can-you-survive-without-water-2014-5?IR=T

2. Microsoft Encarta. (2008). *Fasting.* Retrieved from Microsoft Student 2008 [DVD]Redmond, WA: Microsoft Corporation, 2007

3. Harvard T.H. Chan School of Public Health. (2017). *Manipulating mitochondrial networks could promote healthy aging.* Retrieved from https://medicalxpress.com/news/2017-10-mitochondrial-networks-healthy-aging.html

4. Bernstein, R. (2018). *What foods to eat on omad and what not to.* Retrieved from http://siimland.com/what-foods-to-eat-on-omad/

5. Bhatia, T. (2017). *Water fasting has become super trendy, but is it powerfully healing – or really dangerous?* Retrieved from https://www.mindbodygreen.com/articles/is-

water-fasting-safe-or-healthy

6. Mayo Clinic. (2017). Water: How much should you drink every day? Retrieved from https://www.mayoclinic.org/healthy-lifestyle/nutrition-and-healthy-eating/in-depth/water/art-20044256

7. Fung, J. (2016). *How does fasting affect your brain?* Retrieved from https://www.dietdoctor.com/fasting-affect-brain

8. Science Direct. (2014). *Intermittent fasting vs daily calorie restriction for type 2 diabetes prevention: a review of human findings.* Retrieved from https://www.sciencedirect.com/science/article/pii/S193152441400200X

9. Kettle and Fire. (2018). *Intermittent fasting for women: your complete guide.* Retrieved from https://blog.kettleandfire.com/intermittent-fasting-for-women/

10. Kumar S., Kaur, G. (2013). Intermittent fasting dietary restriction regimen negatively influences reproduction in young rats: A study of hypothalamo-hypophysial-gonadal axis. Retrieved from PLoS ONE 8(1): e52416. https://doi.org/10.1371/journal.pone.0052416

11. American Journal of Managed Care. (2013). *Targeting insulin resistance: The ongoing paradigm shift in diabetes prevention.* Retr Retrieved from http://www.ajmc.com/journals/evidence-based-diabetes-management/2013/2013-1-vol19-sp2/targeting-insulin-resistance-the-ongoing-paradigm-shift-in-diabetes-prevention

12. Rowland, J. (2017). *Signs of Insulin Resistance.* Retrieved from https://www.healthline.com/health/diabetes/insulin-resistance-symptoms

13. Broussard. (2015). Sleep deprivation and fat feeding may reduce insulin action by similar mechanistic pathways. Retrieved from http://www.obesity.org/news/press-releases/one-night-of-poor-sleep-could-equal-six-months-on-a-high-fat-diet

14. US National Library of Medicine. (2011). *Intermittent versus daily calorie restriction: which diet regimen is more effective for weight loss?* Retrieved from https://www.ncbi.nlm.nih.gov/pubmed/21410865

15. US National Library of Medicine. (2013). *Effects of increased meal frequency on fat oxidation and perceived hunger* Retrieved from

https://www.ncbi.nlm.nih.gov/pmc/articles/
PMC4391809/

16. US National Library of Medicine. (2008). *Neuroprotective and disease-modifying effects of the ketogenic diet.* Retrieved from https://www.ncbi.nlm.nih.gov/pmc/articles/ PMC2367001/

17. US National Library of Medicine. (2013). *Beyond weight loss: a review of the therapeutic uses of very-low-carbohydrate (ketogenic) diets.* Retrieved from https://www.ncbi.nlm.nih.gov/pmc/articles/ PMC3826507/

18. Medical Xpress. (2009). *Scientists discover hunger's timekeeper.* Retrieved from https://medicalxpress.com/news/2009-08-scientists-hunger-timekeeper.html#jCp

19. Gustin, A. (2018). Managing Fasting Ketosis: Common signs of ketosis from fasting. Retrieved from https://perfectketo.com/fasting-ketosis-symptoms/

20. Mayo Clinic. (2018). Constipation. Retrieved from https://www.mayoclinic.org/diseases-conditions/constipation/symptoms-causes/syc-20354253

21. US National Library of Medicine. (2010). *Ketogenic diet for treatment of epilepsy.*

Retrieved from
https://www.ncbi.nlm.nih.gov/pmc/articles/
PMC2902940/

22. US National Library of Medicine. (2002).
*Breath acetone is a reliable indicator of
ketosis in adults consuming ketogenic meals*.
Retrieved from
https://www.ncbi.nlm.nih.gov/pubmed/1208
1817

23. US National Library of Medicine. (2017).
*Frequency of consuming foods predicts
changes in cravings for those foods during
weight loss: The pounds lost study*. Retrieved
from
https://www.ncbi.nlm.nih.gov/pubmed/2861
8170

24. DeFazio, L. (2017). *There's a more effective
way to curb your cravings than 'enjoying in
moderation* 'Retrieved from
https://www.womenshealthmag.com/weight-
loss/a19940738/curb-food-cravings/

25. US National Library of Medicine. (2017). *Do
disinhibited eaters pay increased attention to
food cues?* Retrieved from
https://www.ncbi.nlm.nih.gov/pubmed/2769
3488

26. British Journal of Nutrition (2008). *How
does food-cue exposure lead to larger meal*

sizes? Retrieved from
https://www.cambridge.org/core/journals/br
itish-journal-of-nutrition/article/how-does-
food-cue-exposure-lead-to-larger-meal-
sizes/03DCA1B1EA16AD75BE809F1B3075E3
B4#

27. Science Direct. (2011). *The relationship between reward contingency and attention to conditioned food cues.*Retrieved from https://www.sciencedirect.com/science/articl e/pii/S0195666311004259

28. Plos One. (2014). *Startling sweet temptations: Hedonic chocolate deprivation modulates experience, eating behavior, and eyeblink startle.* Retrieved from http://journals.plos.org/plosone/article?id=1 0.1371/journal.pone.0085679

29. US National Library of Medicine. (2008). *Resisting temptation: effects of exposure to a forbidden food on eating behaviour.* Retrieved from https://www.ncbi.nlm.nih.gov/pubmed/1834 2989

30. Selig, M. (2011). *Beware the "what-the-hell effect," especially on holidays!* Retrieved from https://www.psychologytoday.com/blog/cha ngepower/201111/beware-the-what-the-hell- effect-especially-holidays

31. Psychology & Health. (2015). *Associating a prototypical forbidden food item with guilt or celebration: Relationships with indicators of (un)healthy eating and the moderating role of stress and depressive symptoms.*Retrieved from http://www.tandfonline.com/doi/full/10.108 0/08870446.2014.960414?scroll=top&needA ccess=true

32. Freedhoff, Y. (2013).*Why is everyone always giving my kids junk food?* Retrieved from https://health.usnews.com/health-news/blogs/eat-run/2013/02/20/why-is-everyone-always-giving-my-kids-junk-food

33. Bullet Proof. (2018). Glow from the inside out: Autophagy and women – Naomi Whittel #477. Retrieved from https://blog.bulletproof.com/naomi-whittel/

34. Newcastle University. (2018). *How did we evolve to live longer?* Retrieved from https://www.ncl.ac.uk/press/articles/archive /2018/01/howdidweevolvetolivelonger/

35. Bullet Proof. (2018). *Forget juice cleanses. autophagy is the real way to detox your body*. Retrieved from https://blog.bulletproof.com/autophagy-for-longevity-detoxification/#ref-1

36. US National Library of Medicine. (2009).

Starving neurons show sex difference in autophagy. Retrieved from https://www.ncbi.nlm.nih.gov/pmc/articles/PMC2629091/

37. Journal of Cardiovascular Translational Research. (2014). *The role of sex differences in autophagy in the heart during coxsackievirus b3-induced myocarditis.* Retrieved from https://link.springer.com/article/10.1007/s1 2265-013-9525-5

38. Sonpal, N. (2018). *How to exercise safely during intermittent fasting.* Retrieved from https://www.healthline.com/health/how-to-exercise-safely-intermittent-fasting#1

39. Fung, J. (2017). Fasting and Muscle Mass. Retrieved from https://www.dietdoctor.com/fasting-muscle-mass

40. US National Library of Medicine. (2011).*The protein-retaining effects of growth hormone during fasting involve inhibition of muscle-protein breakdown.* Retrieved from https://www.ncbi.nlm.nih.gov/pubmed/1114 7801

41. Mercola, J. (2013). *Should you eat before exercise?* Retrieved from https://fitness.mercola.com/sites/fitness/arc

hive/2013/09/13/eating-before-exercise.aspx

42. Mercola, J. (2011). *The exercise mistake which makes you age faster*. Retrieved from https://articles.mercola.com/sites/articles/archive/2011/06/19/innovative-revolutionary-program-to-keep-your-body-biologically-young.aspx

www.ingramcontent.com/pod-product-compliance
Lightning Source LLC
Chambersburg PA
CBHW050728030426
42336CB00012B/1467